8268 · 610-73 WRI ✓

MY PATIENT – MY NURSE

8268

MY PATIENT – MY NURSE

Second Edition

Stephen G Wright
MBE, RGN, DipN, RCNT,
DANS, RNT, MSc, FRCN

formerly Consultant Nurse, Nursing Development Unit
(Care of the Elderly), Tameside General Hospital
and currently Director, The European Nursing
Development Agency, Tameside

with six contributors

SCUTARI PRESS
London

Scutari Press 1994

A division of Scutari Projects Ltd, the publishing company of the Royal College of Nursing, London.

First published 1994

British Library Cataloguing in Publication Data

Wright, Stephen G.
  My Patient – My Nurse: Guide to Primary
  Nursing. – 2Rev.ed
  I. Title
  610.73
  ISBN 1–871364–94–9

Typeset, printed and bound by The Alden Press

Contents

To
the patients and staff
of the
Nursing Development Unit

and

to a very special nurse
and dear friend
Marie Manthey

Contributors

I am grateful to all my colleagues for the comments and help given in the writing of this text. It was through our experiences and discussions of primary nursing that the idea for the book originated.

Apart from contributing in a general sense to the examples throughout this text, each of my colleagues from the Nursing Development Unit (NDU) provided detailed work to enable me to write certain specific sections:

Susan Archer, RGN, RM (formerly Night Sister in the NDU) on the role of night staff (Chapter 3);

Philip Gartside, RGN (Charge Nurse and Senior Primary Nurse in the NDU) on the various roles in primary nursing (Chapters 3 and 4);

Nasrin Khadim, RGN, FETC (formerly Ward Sister in the NDU and currently Clinical Nurse Specialist) on the setting up of primary nursing and the involvement of the teacher (Chapters 4 and 5);

Elsie Purdy, RGN (formerly Senior Nurse Manager in the NDU and now retired) on the role of the nurse manager (Chapter 5);

Mary Underwood (Care Assistant in the NDU) on the role of the care assistant in the team (Chapter 3);

Gillian Wills, RGN, SEN, FETC (Primary Nurse in the NDU) on organisational matters and evaluation (Chapters 4 and 6).

Acknowledgements

The authors would like to thank the following for their help:

Mr R Butterworth, Unit General Manager, and Mr M L Johnson, Assistant Unit General Manager, for their continuing support in enabling it all to happen and for their kind permission to reproduce the job descriptions in the Appendix.

Mr R Davenport, Unit General Manager when the Nursing Development Unit was created, Mr W A Bamber, also a former Unit General Manager, and the senior medical staff, Dr M A Matin, Dr A H Wan, Dr O M P Jolobe and Dr Sil, for their encouragement of nursing.

Mr T W Fisher, OBE, Assistant General Manager (Quality Assurance) and Chief Nurse Adviser, for his interest and support.

Special thanks must also go to Mrs Irene Hill, Secretary, for assistance above and beyond the call of duty, and to Mr Ian Webster and Mrs M McDermott for their invaluable help and many cups of tea.

The Tameside Nursing Development Unit and the European Nursing Development Agency images and logos were designed by Total Concept Design (UK) Ltd, Manchester.

Foreword

'Primary nursing is more than a simple way of organising
nurses; it is a voyage into nursing's little-explored territories, a journey into a new reality.' So claim Steve Wright
and his colleagues in this splendidly readable book. And
they invite their readers to enter, with them, into the
world of primary nursing. In so doing, they show how the
vision of primary nursing transforms the understanding of
the nature of nursing and also how primary nursing can be
achieved in very practical ways.

The essence of primary nursing is encapsulated in the
concepts of fellowship and companionship. Its purpose is
to enable each patient to relate to 'my nurse' and each
nurse to develop a special relationship with 'my patient'.
Nurse and patient accompany each other during the
patient's voyage through illness, dependency, recovery –
or the valley of the shadow of death. The opportunity that
primary nursing provides for nurses and patients to
develop this deep companionship is a vital factor in the
healing potential inherent in nursing.

Steve Wright and his colleagues move on from a convincing general discussion of the value of primary nursing
to a detailed and equally convincing discussion of practicalities. They provide answers to some of the most
worrying questions that confront nurses who might want
to adopt primary nursing. In so doing, they share some of
the problems they have experienced and the solutions they
have found, with regard to issues such as the role of the
ward sister/charge nurse, the contribution of enrolled
nurses, night duty and access to nursing notes.

The authors finish with the challenge 'Pursue your

vision!' Having read this book, and seen this vision in practice in their unit, I hope that many nurses will rise to the challenge, share the vision and achieve the reality, for their own benefit and, ultimately all-important, for the benefit of their patients.

Baroness Cox of Queensbury,
BSc(Soc), MSc(Econ), RGN, FRCN

Preface to the First Edition

The Nursing Development Unit in the Care of the Elderly Unit at Tameside General Hospital was formally set up in 1986. It was the culmination of many years of previous work, aimed at producing change in nursing practice for the older patient. From the start, it was one of our goals to implement primary nursing – not just as a means of organising care, but as part of the whole way in which we think about nursing and how it should be practised.

Since those early days, almost 10 years ago, we have witnessed the entry of primary nursing into the debating forum of nursing and its growth in many sections of health care. Many nurses have visited the unit to find out about primary nursing, or have quizzed the staff at various courses and conferences as to how it might be done.

Inevitably, the concerns and questions of many nurses proved to be the same: How many staff do you need? What about the doctors? Can the enrolled nurse be a primary nurse? What can the manager do? and so on, and so on.

This book is in part a response to those uncertainties. We have tried to produce very much a 'how to do it' text that will answer many of those questions and deal with the practicalities of primary nursing in the everyday world of the nurse. At the same time, we hope to share with the reader a vision of what primary nursing might be, which is more than a mere system to deploy nurses differently. Aiming for the goal of primary nursing brings with it a wholesale reappraisal of what nursing is and how nurses should work with each other, their patients, colleagues, visitors and other carers.

We have tried to fill this book with our own experiences

and views, and, in so doing, we hope that you, the reader, whether doubtful or enthusiastic, will enhance your own knowledge of primary nursing. Perhaps if you are just beginning the journey towards primary nursing, you will find it less fraught with difficulties, avoid some of the pitfalls and reach your destination sooner if you are armed with the knowledge of how others have travelled the path before. It is our experience and our belief that primary nursing can help nurses do their job better, with benefit to both patients and themselves, and this, after all, is what matters.

Throughout the text the word 'patient' is used for simplicity. 'Client', 'resident', or any other word the reader is familiar with for the recipient of care, is equally applicable.

Steve Wright and colleagues
December 1988

Preface to the Second Edition

Since my colleagues and I put together the first edition, so much has changed in the world of nursing. The whole basis of health care provision in the UK has been challenged and reforms continue apace. In Eastern and Central Europe, political changes of gigantic proportions have swept away old certainties. Across the world whole societies are in flux as political and economic pressures shake established systems.

The pace of change has accelerated as Toffler (1973) predicted that it would. Nurses and nursing have felt threatened and victimised or have risen to explore new opportunities to expand their roles.

Yet in the midst of all this, primary nursing has continued to expand not only in the UK but internationally. As 12 000 nurses gathered in Madrid for the 1993 International Congress of Nurses, it became clear from the many presentations that primary nursing had strengthened its position as an international phenomenon. It continues to increase its influence not only on the delivery of patient care, but also on the way nurses and nursing are growing and nurses are seeing their work and themselves within the scheme of things.

Meanwhile, the Tameside NDU continues to prosper, and, like everyone else, has had to respond to the many changes which confront it. The role of primary nursing within the NDU remains one of its principal facets – and the DNU has played its part well in helping to disseminate ideas both in the UK and internationally. This second edition provides an opportunity to update the text with recent events, writings and research. I have added many new references, as well as additional work on, for example, support worker roles, the expansion of primary nursing, the relationship to the 'named nurse' concept and so on. I have updated some sections in the light of developments in the Tameside unit, and considerably extended many others. More questions and responses have been added, for example, to what was the original 'twenty questions' chapter.

I hope the reader finds this revised work helpful. Much of it has been possible with the comments, questions and suggestions that have come forward from hundreds of nurses over the years. It seems that despite criticisms, conflicts and challenges, primary nursing has followed my predicted course – one of inexorable growth.

Stephen G Wright, MBE, RGN, DipN,
RCNT, DANS, RNT, MSc, FRCN
Director, TENDA
August 1993

'How do you expect us to fly as you fly?',
came another voice. 'You are special and
gifted and divine, above other birds.'

Look at Fletcher! Lowell! Charles-Rowland!
Are they also special and gifted and divine?
No more than you are, no more than I am.
The only difference, the very only one,
is that they have begun to understand what
they really are and have begun to practise it.

Richard Bach
Jonathan Livingston Seagull

CHAPTER 1

An Introduction to Primary Nursing

Fellowship is heaven, and lack of fellowship is hell;
Fellowship is life, and the lack of fellowship death;
and the deeds that ye do upon the earth, it is for
fellowship's sake that ye do them.

William Morris
The Dream of John Bull

Traditional views of the history of nursing tend to follow a very typical model. Nursing is seen as constantly progressing, marching forward in time, while forever improving, overcoming great odds and striving towards excellence.

A closer examination of the past might raise a few questions over this view. Whole forests must have been felled to produce the paper for a veritable mountain of reports, research documents and royal commissions. They span many decades and indicate that in fact all is not well with nursing, nor has it been for some time. There are many deep-rooted problems in nursing; much does not appear to have changed fundamentally over the years.

Two principal perspectives seem to emerge – those of the patient and of the nurse.

The Patient's View

Much recent work (e.g. Henderson, 1980; Lanara, 1981; Health Service Ombudsman 1986–1993; Pearson, 1988a, b) illustrates a continued dissatisfaction of patients with the quality of care which they receive, particularly concerning the quality of the nurse–patient relationship. The Health Service Ombudsman's reports (1986–1993), for example, indicate dissatisfaction with nursing, which has many common threads – failures in communication, uncaring attitudes, inattention to needs – quite apart from failings in expertise associated with many physical tasks such as attention to hygiene or wound care. Pearson (1988a, b) has noted how 'patients themselves agree with the view that nurses are obsessed with the performance of tasks associated with physical care and the support of medical regimes, and that they do not fulfil expectations as the humanisers of the health care systems'. Patients appear to want a positive, healing, helpful relationship with nurses, yet so often nurses are told not to 'get involved' with patients. Nursing, on the contrary, is about being 'involved' with patients, but it is an involvement within defined limits that they seek, a therapeutic relationship for patients that does not harm them while at the same time does not damage or exhaust nurses. Primary nursing is about the redefining of that relationship and the role of the nurse in it. The primary nurse is nothing if not 'involved' with the patient.

The challenge of primary nursing is to overcome these weaknesses. This is not, however, to suggest that nurses should 'throw the baby out with the bathwater'! Nursing has many valuable qualities and these should be cherished and built upon. The call to primary nursing is not to suggest that everything before has been bad – it has not – and that, if we would but implement primary nursing, everything in the future would be perfect – it would not. Rather it is a call to look more closely at what nurses and patients value and to redefine how nurses should think and act in the light of these needs.

Lanara (1981) argues that 'nursing today is at a critical

and, one might say, tragic crossroads. The nurse is better educated, more knowledgeable and more science-orientated. Yet the patient, for all the superb physical and technical improvements in his environment, feels lonely and even abandoned, because nobody cares for him as a person'. Lanara goes on to suggest that for nurses the way forward is to re-examine and define their beliefs, enriching what already exists, to bring about 'the awakening of the spirit of nursing, which, integrated with science and technology, will re-create the living spirit in a matrix of concern'.

Some years ago, I was involved in a survey of patients' and staff opinions on what constituted 'good' nursing (Wright, 1987a). This preliminary work aimed at devising some quality assurance tools. In the survey, nurses tended to see the 'good' nurse as being 'hard working', 'tidy', 'efficient', 'carrying out procedures correctly', and so on.

Interestingly, many of the patients seemed to lay more emphasis on different issues. One patient summed this up quite succinctly. 'Look, it's like this, when I come into your ward, I want to feel the nurse *cares* for me. I'd rather she told me what's going on than keep washing me all the time. When I come through the doors of your ward, I want a nurse who says: "Hello, I'm Nurse so-and-so, I've been expecting you. I'm going to look after you while you're here. If you want to know anything, I'll keep you informed, and your wife too! So first I'll settle you in bed. After that, we'll spend some time together sorting out what we can do to help so you know where you're going"'.

This particular patient went on to describe in graphic detail what the qualities of 'his' nurse should be – informing, teaching, supporting, being 'on his side', involving his family, keeping him safe, and so on. The extraordinary common sense of this patient made me look again at how I and my colleagues projected ourselves, and gave new impetus to our innovations on making care more personal.

Consultant nurse

The Nurse's View

If patients are not always fully satisfied with nursing, then there is also parallel dissatisfaction among nurses. Nurses demonstrate this with their feet, producing an attrition rate so great that nursing must reproduce itself every 10 years simply to keep enough nurses at the bedside (RCN, 1986). Other documents mirror the American experience of the 'Magnet Hospitals' study (McLure el al, 1983), indicating that while nurses' salary levels contribute to the exodus, equally important are high levels of dissatisfaction with the 'climate' (created by negative management attitudes) in which they work, and the sense of powerlessness at being unable to practise nursing in the manner in which they feel they should (Dean, 1988; Price Waterhouse, 1988; Strong and Robinson, 1988).

Movements in the nursing workforce appear to have been affected recently by economic factors and high unemployment levels. Nurses in jobs are tending to remain in them, and there is evidence (RCN, 1993a) not only of a reduction in the number of jobs available to nurses, but also of reduced opportunities for promotion or change of grade. These factors are believed to have contributed even further to declining morale among nurses, especially when they have been accompanied by major organisational change within the National Health Service, and a steady increase in the size of the independent sector. While individuals, professional and service organisations and governments seek to deal with these issues, it also reinforces the need to examine the way nurses work – it is important to deal with concerns about pay and job security, but it is also important to ensure that nursing is carried out in the most efficient and effective ways – ways which also help nurses to feel more satisfied with the work they do.

Primary nursing suggests that nurses should practise with greater professional autonomy. It also opens the way for nurses to achieve job satisfaction by extending their relationship with patients, so that they know they are meeting their needs. Thus, while primary nursing can do little to address itself to nurses' pay, it has the potential to deal with those other dissatisfactions in nurses related to the organisation of care.

PRIMARY NURSING – A HISTORICAL BACKGROUND

To some extent, primary nursing is a return to what Nightingale (1869) defined as her 'case method' approach to nursing – an individual (trained) nurse being responsible for a given group of patients, dealing with a variety of issues related to health, hygiene and family support. While the education (and hence knowledge base) of the Nightingale nurses was not as highly developed as in more recent times (nor was the notion of the 'professional nurse'), there are many commonalities. To that extent, primary nursing might be seen as a return to the case method, a rediscovery perhaps of what is at the heart of nursing.

It is important to remember that the principles of primary nursing have been applied in many sectors of nursing for decades. Much of the current focus on developing primary nursing has related to hospital care. However, many health visitors, community nurses and independent midwives, for example, have continued to practise by having individual caseloads of patients/clients for whom they accept responsibility with a high level of continuity.

Primary nursing (or health visiting or midwifery) has certain principles (q.v.) which enable each practitioner to make explicit the nature of their role and the way they work with their patients or clients.

The post-Nightingale era witnessed a growing hospital base for nursing and the rise of the scientific medical model dominating health care. Shortages of nurses (especially during war time) compounded the problem. The result was the evolution of the 'task-centred' approach to care. Lee (1979) notes how task-centred nursing follows an industrial model, breaking down care into groups of (nursing) tasks carried out by nurses according to skill and status (the 'back round', the 'obs round', the 'toilet round'). Beyers and Philips (1971) note that the 'case method' was 'expensive in terms of professional nursing salaries and impractical for most nursing units'. In part, argues

Menzies (1961), the tasks also became a means of containing anxiety. Unable to cope with the difficulties of working in large bureaucratic organisations and with the stress of dealing with the totality of the patients and their problems, nurses responded, Menzies argues, by dividing aspects of patient care into neat chunks which could be more easily managed. Henderson (1980) suggests that this ultimately proved satisfying to neither patient nor nurse. Both were dehumanised in the process: completing the tasks does not remove the sense of failure on the part of the nurse from seeing how much care has *not* been given, while the patient is short-changed on care which cannot easily be task allocated (e.g. teaching or comforting).

Despite the 'dehumanising' risks associated with task allocation, many nurses appear to have made great efforts to treat patients as human beings. Kindness and comfort can still be relayed in task-allocation settings even though such a system may militate against them. 'Task-allocation' has now almost become a pejorative term in nursing, but it is necessary to be wary of dismissing a mode of practice which has served so many nurses for so many years. To do so is to imply that 'everything was bad' before and, by implication, so were the nurses involved in it. In reality, many nurses appeared to have recognised the flaws in task allocation and sought to deal with them. Some strove to be more humane in their dealings with patients, some would (often surreptitiously) seek to bring more interpersonal skills into their care. (It is often reported in nursing mythology that the nurse who sought to 'get involved' would 'never make a nurse', or the nurse caught sitting and talking with a patient would be asked to 'find some work to do'!) Other nurses, meanwhile, looked to rethinking the way care was organised.

Efforts to break away from the reductionist industrialised approach inherent in task-centred nursing led to developments in team nursing (Waters, 1985) and patient allocation (Marks-Maran, 1978). However, these methods (while seeming to have fewer nurses caring for fewer patients, for large periods of time, and hence making care more personal) are open to abuse. Nurses working in teams still tend to split care into tasks among the team. Patient allocation leaves open the question of the level of expertise of the nurse to whom the patient is allocated (auxiliary? student? trained nurse?) and the length of time of the allocation. Furthermore, accountability and autonomy in both these methods remain unclear.

> We'd organised the ward for a long time on the basis of patient allocation. For us, moving to primary nursing was the next logical step. In that sense, we found that patient allocation was the precursor of primary nursing.
>
> *Ward sister/primary nurse*

To some degree, therefore, the advent of primary nursing may be seen as an evolutionary process (Figure 1.1) with elements of a desire to return to certain earlier values and methods in the organisation of nursing care.

Fig. 1.1 Primary nursing as an evolutionary process

However, it would be a mistake to view these trends as a neat cycle of historical events. The birth of one has not necessarily led to the extinction of the other. All these methods of organising nursing can be found in practice simultaneously in many parts of nursing at present.

It is interesting to note also that the use of primary nursing as a dominant theme in recent years has occurred alongside two other major topics in nursing practice – the nursing process and nursing models. A full explanation of these last two issues is beyond the scope of this text, but it might be useful to examine briefly how they are linked to primary nursing (Figure 1.2).

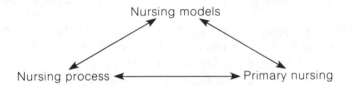

Fig. 1.2   The link between the nursing process, models and primary nursing

NURSING MODELS

Every nurse carries in his or her head an 'image' (Reilly, 1975) of what nursing is. This informal model, the way each nurse thinks about nursing, has important implications, for it determines the way in which the nurse acts out nursing. For example, the nurse's beliefs about the elderly, whether as hopeless cases or as individuals with potential for rehabilitation, will affect the way in which the nurse works with those patients. When nurses start to pool these beliefs, ideas and concepts about what nursing is, they can construct more formal models (Wright, 1986). The next step is then to decide how these are put into practice. If, for example, the notion that care should be 'individualised' is espoused, then how is it done? What is the best method of organisation to make care so personal: patient allocation? task allocation? primary nursing?

NURSING PROCESS

In carrying out nursing, another question arises. How does the nurse decide what help is needed? The nursing process might simply be described as the tool by which nursing is thought through. Thus, by assessing the patients for their needs, deciding what needs to be done (planning) and actually getting on with it (implementing), while at the same time making sure it is effective (evaluating), the 'process cycle' is established.

PRIMARY NURSING

The process of nursing helps us to identify what help is needed. A nursing model may help to define what system is used to identify and plan patient care. Both throw out challenges as the best way to organise care so that the patient's personal needs are met. Primary nursing, as an organisational tool, helps nurses to put into practice some of the beliefs and concepts which underpin their choice of model and to work with patients as individuals whose needs and care can be identified and pursued.

However formal or informal their model of care, primary nurses use this to guide their practice and planning of care so that it is co-ordinated and comprehensive. Primary nursing can therefore be seen as one option for nurses to put their beliefs and ideas about nursing into action, using the nursing process as a basis for working out the patient's care. Models, process and primary nursing are therefore all intimately linked (Figure 1.2), and it is the practice upon which the contributors to this book have based their work.

The Rise of Primary Nursing

Some recent surveys have suggested that, in hospitals at least (both public and independent), there has been a steady increase in the use of primary nursing in the UK. Studies carried out by the Audit Commission (1991) and the Institute of Manpower Studies (1992) indicate similar trends. In 1981, about 75% of hospital nursing settings appear to have been using task allocation as a means of organising care. A decade later, nursing seemed to have transformed itself. Only about 10% were still using task allocation, while primary nursing (less than 1% in 1981) had increased to 16%. Patient allocation and team nursing were each being applied in about one-third of the remaining settings.

The significance of this change should not be under-estimated. It represents a huge shift in working patterns for many thousands of nurses in only 10 years. While there are many pressure groupings and influential individuals in nursing, such a change cannot be attributed to these alone. Furthermore, this appears very much to have been a practice-led phenomenon, refuting the view held by some (Finch, 1991) that primary nursing has been adopted by 'superior' nurses in 'superior' settings. Primary nursing has indeed become quite commonplace. That it has done so is largely attributable to thousands of nurses around the country who have quietly and purposefully implemented it.

Many questions could be asked about these and similar surveys, not least how the concepts of team and primary nursing, for example, were being defined. Because of lack of clarity of definition (or to create a good impression) perhaps some nurses indicated that they were primary nursing when team nursing was the case, and so on. However, leaving these views aside, British nursing, within a decade, does appear to have undergone a startling transformation in terms of its dominant methods of organisation.

The trend towards primary nursing appears to be unabated. There has been a huge proliferation of litera-ture, conferences and study days on the subject. Teaching packages (Perera and Miller, 1993) and courses have been offered (Turnock, 1990); in one instance, a course has been developed to diploma level (Wade, 1992).

Primary nursing appears to have been applied to every conceivable nursing setting (Hiscox, 1990; Wicker, 1990; Chilton, 1991; Marlow, 1991; Ersser and Tutton, 1991;

Black, 1992; Wright, 1993, for example), reinforced by the work of the King's Fund Centre and its Primary Nursing Network and nursing development programmes. The network issued its own newsletter, detailing the experiences of nurses across the country from many different specialities. Local special interest groups on the subject are also a common phenomenon.

The Audit Commission (1992) went on to endorse strongly the spread of primary nursing as the preferred method of organising high quality patient care. In building on the Strategy for Nursing (DoH, 1989), the 'Vision for the Future' (NHSME, 1993) sees primary nursing as a principal platform to develop the 'named nurse' approach. The Patient's Charter (DoH, 1991) for the first time made explicit that patients should have a 'named qualified nurse, midwife or health visitor responsible for your nursing or midwifery care'. Subsequent guidance (NHSME, 1992; Wright, 1993) specified the organisational methods which could be used to achieve this, including primary nursing as a method of choice. In an early response to the 'named nurse' policy, Hancock (1991a) saw primary nursing as the 'clearest expression' of the named nurse concept – superior to other methods such as team nursing or patient allocation.

The relationship between primary nursing and named nursing is very close, and will be pursued further in Chapter 4. Meanwhile it is worth raising the questions at this stage of how far such a high profile and wide endorsement is helpful to nurses in practice, and whether or not changing an organisational method *necessarily* means that the quality of care improves. In relation to the former, it may mean that some nurses find themselves under pressure to implement primary nursing in a 'top down' fashion – in order to meet management or organisational objectives. Resistance to change may be increased as a result, or the approach is never really adopted wholeheartedly because nurses do not 'own' the changes or understand the true nature of primary nursing. In Chapter 2, more attention is given to appropriate patterns of change in primary nursing.

Changing an organisational method of care is no guarantee that care will improve. The relationship between the two is an assumed one. Thus, if task allocation is dissatisfying to patients and nurses, then logic suggests that changing to a more patient-centred approach to care, e.g. primary nursing, should remove these dissatisfactions and may produce other improvements. Other factors, however, appear to be significant, not least the nature of the nurse–patient relationship, the way the nurse works with the patient and the ability of the nurse to transfer the philosophical side of primary nursing (based on values related to the individual worth of each patient, the potential of nursing as a therapeutic force and so on). These issues will be dealt with in more detail in Chapter 3.

PRIMARY NURSING AS A CROSS-CULTURAL PROCESS

While many of the earlier writings on primary nursing (Hall, 1969; Manthey, 1970, 1973) have their origins in the USA, it should be emphasised that developments in primary nursing have taken place across the world. In that sense, it should be seen not as an import from one nation, but rather as a concurrent transcultural process. Descriptions and evaluations of primary nursing have emerged, for example, from:

- Australia (Watson, 1978)
- Japan (Otoya, 1979; Toshiko, 1993)
- UK (Lee, 1979; Sparrow, 1986)
- Norway (Aschjem et al, 1979)
- Belgium (Blanpain, 1976)
- The Netherlands (Van Eindhoven, 1979)
- Canada (Medaglia, 1978)
- Switzerland (Roth, 1993)
- Finland (Karpov, 1991)
- Taiwan (Ku, 1993)

Manthey (1970) appears to have been the progenitor of the term 'primary nursing' but, in doing so, she seems to have focused on an idea with international implications. Nurses across the globe seem to share common concerns, goals and hopes in their desire to reaffirm nursing as a patient-centred practice. Primary nursing taps that transcultural nursing desire.

PRIMARY NURSING DEFINED

While patient allocation and the case method, for example, have in some ways offered directions for more personal care, they do not address themselves sufficiently to the principles of professional practice, and accountability or the degrees of knowledge and skill which underpin them. Indeed, Hall (1969) derides team or task nursing as 'getting through the work' and the mark of a 'trade', not a profession, and thus a disservice to the patient. Patient allocation may be applied, for example, on an ad hoc basis and any grade of nurse might be used (Wright, 1987b), while the older case method relied upon the limited vision of the nurse's role available at the time (a weaker knowledge base and subservience to medical practice). The 'case method' approach in modern nursing, for example in health visiting, now tends to be used almost synonymously with primary nursing.

As Hegyvary (1982) notes, primary nursing 'is both a philosophy of care and an organisational design. It is not simply a way of assigning nurses to patients, but rather a view of nursing as a professional, patient-centred practice'. Manthey (1980) writes of the development of the 'my nurse' concept and provides one of the best definitions of primary nursing: 'The nursing care of a specific patient is under the continuous guidance of one nurse from admission through to discharge. One nurse on each shift provides total care for the same group of patients day after day. Round the clock care is co-ordinated for each patient by the nurse designated as the primary nurse for that patient'. The implications of putting into practice the above statement are profound, not only for the professionalisation of nursing and the effects on the quality of patient care, but also for the wider organisations and society in which the nurse works.

While Hall (1969) has dismissed non-primary nursing as having the characteristics of a 'trade', Manthey (1980) has referred to other forms as an attempt to 'deprofessionalise' nursing. Breaking down nursing into simple components, it is argued, emphasises a bureaucratic organisation of nursing, which does little to enhance the status of, and the satisfaction with, nursing, of both nurses and patients.

Rotkontch (1979) has argued that the term 'primary nursing' should not be used because of possible confusion with primary care. She regards the term 'professional nursing practice' as adequate. Hegyvary notes that these terms can become confusing because of over-use and misuse. Primary nursing, however, must be seen as a distinct entity. A nurse in the community as part of a primary care team (i.e. promoting health outside the hospital setting) may be practising in either a task-centred or primary nursing way. 'Nursing is a profession only to the extent to which nursing performs professional roles; merely performing tasks or delegating everything to others does not meet the criteria [for professional nursing] . . . nor does holding the title "professional nurse" ensure that the nurse performs at a professional level' (Hegyvary, 1982). The issue of nursing as a profession is debatable, but primary nursing offers a professional model (see Chapter 6) which nurses can follow because it contains the following basic ingredients for professional practice:

- *Accountability.* The primary nurse is answerable for the nursing care of the patient or family 24 hours a day, while in his or her care, whether in hospital or the community.
- *Autonomy.* In the mode of 'professional self-governance', the primary nurse has the authority, and acts on it, to make decisions about the patient's, or family's, nursing care.
- *Co-ordination.* A smooth flow of nursing care exists from shift to shift with direct communication from care-giver to care-giver.

• *Comprehensiveness.* Each care-giver gives all the nursing care required during the course of a shift (sometimes called 'total patient care').

Primary nursing is essentially the function of the 'primary (registered) nurse'. In his/her absence, 'associate' nurses take over the nursing care, but they remain responsible to the primary nurse for carrying out the agreed plan of care or revising it as conditions change.

It is acknowledged (Manthey, 1980) that the above four elements are not always achievable absolutely in every situation, but it is argued that they 'set the standards or goals for defining the essence of primary nursing'. She notes how much depends on the abilities of the nurse and the nature of the organisational structure to achieve success. She comments: 'Primary nursing does not define or guarantee the quality of nursing care. As a system, it *facilitates* a very high level of quality by enabling and empowering individuals to perform at their maximum capacity' (Manthey, 1980). Thus, to modify Nightingale's (1869) earlier words defining nursing ('putting the patient in the best position for nature to act'), primary nursing puts the nurses in the best position for nursing to act.

Primary nursing is a challenge to nurses. It opens a 'can of worms', letting loose many aspects of nursing that they may have chosen to hide from or ignore. Not every nurse will wish to be, or can be, a primary nurse, and perhaps many would wish to retreat when faced with the enormity of the implications. How far can the nurse be accountable? What will the nature of the relationship with the patients be, and how can it be managed? What sort of education or management is needed to foster primary nursing? How can it be organised? How will relationships with colleagues be affected? Who will be the primary nurse?

Primary nursing is a call to nurses to come out of their shells, to assert themselves and to seek answers to questions like these. The following chapters of this book will address themselves to these issues – and more.

Primary nursing means change, and, faced with the seeming enormity of the task, it is little wonder that many nurses might resist and retreat. Perhaps, after all, it would be better to keep things as they are and cloak the potential of nursing in the mantle of others (let the doctor or the sister tell me what to do!). As Kafka (1916) succinctly points out, 'sometimes it is safer to be in chains than to be free'. Primary nursing is more than a simple way of organising nurses; it is a voyage into nursing's little-explored territories, a journey into a new reality.

CHAPTER 2

Changing to Primary Nursing

Hos successus alit possunt
quia posse videntur

Success nourished them; they seemed
to be able, and so they were able

Virgil
The Aeneid

To develop primary nursing implies, inevitably, that things
must change. If primary nursing is different from the status
quo, there will be movement away from something (the way
we always did things) towards something (our new way of
doing things). Very often in nursing there has been a
tendency to implement change by forcing it through, using
a 'top-down' power–coercive approach, i.e. orders passed
down through the hierarchy. Such an approach is fatally
flawed, for staff forced into change will usually invent all
manner of ways to resist, distort or disrupt the change.
This happened in many parts of the UK with the implementation of the nursing process.

Another strategy is to use the 'hero-innovator' model
(Georgiades and Phillimore, 1975), tapping the skills of
particular energetic and charismatic leaders who attempt
to lead the staff into change, only to burn out, leaving the
change to collapse and return to the old order when they
have gone (and, in so doing, prove the doubters right that

the change would never work anyway!). It is equally difficult to implement change when impetus comes from only
one or two staff in a particular setting, or when the
enthusiast does not have the power and control to change
things.

I was really sold on primary nursing as soon as I read about it, and the
conference just filled me with more enthusiasm. But where do I start? – I'm
only the enrolled nurse. The charge nurse isn't going to listen to me, and
the manager doesn't like anything that rocks the boat.

After a while, I got the impression that I was on my own in this. I began
to feel that people were leaving the clinic early to go on their rounds just to
avoid talking to me about the subject.

Enrolled nurse (community)

The theory and application of change are complex subjects, which it is beyond the scope of this text to explore in
full. British texts are now emerging (Pearson, 1992; Wright,
1989) that suggest ways in which nurses at clinical level
can change practice. Some of the salient points can be
brought together to form a change strategy to help to ease
the path through the change process.

A CHANGE STRATEGY

The move towards primary nursing needs to go hand in
hand with a change strategy – planning the change as
much as possible to minimise conflicts and promote progress and co-operation.

Salvage (1988a) comments that 'shock, withdrawal and
apathy' are among the responses that managers and
colleagues can feel when the nurse 'breezes in with her
bright new idea. To what extent are they inevitable aspects
of human behaviour and to what extent can they be
anticipated and outwitted?' It seems that part of the solut-
ion is to plan the change. This is supported by Pearson and
Vaughan (1986), who contend that 'some changes occur
because of things around us, but most changes cannot
effectively occur without being planned. Planned change is

inevitably easier to manage than change which is imposed, haphazard or misunderstood!'.

Thus a nursing process type of problem-solving approach can be helpful as part of an overall strategy. This involves identifying all the various facets of a situation and working out how to overcome them (assessing and planning). For example: Are there key people who need to be convinced? What information is needed? What resources are required? and so on. Then a gradual implementation of the plan takes place, with careful monitoring and evaluation to determine how it is working. In practice, however, the change process is rarely so linear, and a successful change programme requires an immense amount of flexibility to take into account numerous other factors. Change is invariably 'messy'.

Turrill (1985) suggests that some of these other factors in the plan should include the following:

- *Getting people together to agree the core purpose of the organisation:* e.g. does primary nursing fit in with the goals of the ward or unit to make care individualised?
- *Sharing a vision of a better future.* Primary nursing requires its advocates to have that vision, knowing that it cannot be achieved overnight, but seeing the goal always on the horizon and working towards it. Lasting change will not occur unless a critical core of the staff in a given setting shares the same vision and is willing to work towards it.

Most of the staff were doubtful or downright difficult, but it only took the few of us. Just three of us out of the whole ward shared the same wishes, but we persisted. We learnt, we worked at it, eventually we won through.

Primary nurse

- *Setting the working principles.* Thus, in the case of primary nursing, the ground rules need to be laid, perhaps identifying clearly who does what within the team, where each member's responsibilities lie, and reaching agreements on how conflicts will be dealt with.

- *Mapping the environment:* identifying the implications for other individuals and groups, and how these might be dealt with, e.g. how will the doctors be approached on this? What do the other disciplines, relatives, patients and colleagues need to know? This includes working out in advance how to respond to them.
- *Transition management:* managing the problems that occur between the start and finish lines of the change. The task that each is required to do can be clearly spelt out, as well as what resources are needed, e.g. new forms of nursing documentation.
- *Resistance reduction.* Copious two-way communication is necessary so that the team have a chance to explain and explore their feelings, question, clarify and seek information. Involving other groups in the change, listening to their point of view and engaging their support help to reduce resistance.

Because we were working more flexibly, we had some problems with the portering staff. They were getting angry because we were disrupting their schedule for collecting the meal trolleys. We invited them to some of the ward meetings and introduced them to patients who said how much better things were. When they (the porters) felt part of it, when they saw what we were doing was helping patients, they understood and looked at their own way of doing things so that they could help us.

Senior primary nurse/charge nurse

- *Seeking commitment.* Identifying key groups and indi–viduals and devising non-threatening ways of winning them over helps to draw them into the change process.

It was really the nursing officer who was pushing for it. She thought primary nursing was a great idea, but we weren't so sure. We were impressed, though, when she joined us on the ward and worked as part of the team, showing us not only how it could be done but that it was possible, drawing more of us into it. She was there as our example, ready with the facts and the support.

Associate nurse

Changing anything in nursing is no doubt easier if there is a culture of innovation. If the setting has a climate that encourages change and sees it as part of normal day-to-day work, change is very much easier. Much of the responsibility for this lies in the hands of the nurse manager, and this will be dealt with later in Chapter 5. Manthey (1980) suggests that it may take many years for change to filter throughout the organisation, but this can be aided by total organisational commitment to the change. Setting up support groups and steering committees including all levels of staff can help to plan the changes and provide the thrust to keep the plans moving forward.

Other dimensions of a change strategy are explained by Ottoway (1976, 1980) and have been developed to apply to nursing settings (Wright, 1989; Pearson, 1992). Some of the main points (Figure 2.1) include the following:

- *The presence of a change agent.* A change agent is a key person knowledgeable in the subject and in how to

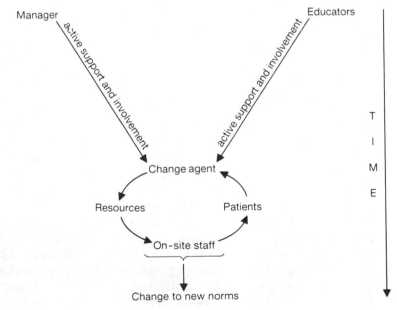

Fig. 2.1 Change strategy

change things. It is better if the change agent works on
site, with the staff, involved in their day-to-day
practice. The position in the system is also important,
i.e. changing practice on a particular unit is easier if
the designated change agents have more control
because they are 'clinical leaders' (e.g. ward sister or
charge nurse) in the organisation. Where nursing
practice is changing, it is particularly helpful if the
change agent has the credibility of being a practising
nurse working with the staff. Managers and teachers
who stand outside the organisation will find that
getting staff to accept change will be more difficult.

- *Managers and educators*, where they are part of the
clinical team, have a crucial part to play in giving
support and guidance, staff counselling and supplying
information and resources. If support of either of these
groups is lacking, the change process will be hindered
that much more.

- The *on-site staff* must be involved in the change process,
whatever their status or role. For the change to be
effective and long lasting, the new norms must be
'owned' by the staff. Ownership, through involvement
in the decision-making process, taking account of views
and using suggestions, is essential for new behaviours
to be implemented. This 'bottom-up' approach ensures
staff participation and the generation of change at
clinical level. The change agent's role and skills here
are very important in guiding and encouraging this
process, without seeming to dominate and control.
Otherwise the staff will perceive it as a 'top-down'
process, merely responding to orders. There is then a
risk, if the change agent leaves or is absent, that the
on-site staff will revert to the old norms.

- *Resources*. These include the provision of equipment
and information and reviewing the number and skill
mix of the staff (see 'The Manager's Role' in Chapter 5).
If the staff are not adequately resourced to pursue the
changes, they may suffer guilt through failure, reject
the changes or exhaust themselves in an effort to keep
the changes going. Nurses are often exhorted to

change, yet not always given the wherewithal to do it. It is futile, for example, to embark upon primary nursing unless there is a concurrent commitment to examine, and change where necessary, the number and mix of staff.

> I was told I could get on with primary nursing provided I made do with what I'd got. I didn't want more staff, just a review of the existing workforce. There are only three trained staff in this ward. The rest are auxiliaries. It's no use telling me I can change things, and then do nothing to help me do it.
>
> *Ward sister*

- *Patients.* If primary nursing is deemed to help patients, then they can and must be involved in the change towards it. More details of how this can be done appear in Chapter 4.
- *Time.* Dealing with the problems that arise, preparing the ground and seeing these changes through can take a long time. Often it is the preparatory work that takes the longest.

> We've had many visitors come to the unit to learn about primary nursing. Some of them, I felt, assumed they could pick up a few facts and implement it the next day. Hopefully, by the time we had related our experiences and gone through all the implications, they've been a little more realistic. I hope we haven't put them off, but enthusiasm needs to be tempered with practicality. Here, it took us the best part of 4 years before we really made headway. In that time, we had to attend to a lot of things to make care more personal, and we had to work with the managers to look at the mix of staff and change it. Originally about 80% of the workforce were nursing auxiliaries. You can't do primary nursing with that. Now, on average, it's been revised to about 65% trained staff. The whole place had to change. It was wheels within wheels, because we couldn't have recruited the trained staff unless we'd done something about the image of the care of the elderly to attract the staff in the first place. We had to work towards primary nursing, passing through patient allocation first. Some people say primary nursing is easier in the care of the elderly − they should try it! Every place has its difficulties; they are just different difficulties in different places.
>
> *Consultant nurse*

Thus it can take many years for the groundwork to be done so that a setting becomes 'ripe' for primary nursing. This 'ripeness' is characterised by the shared values of the staff and the readiness to change. However, every setting will be different, and some may have the initial foundations which allow for a very rapid transition. Once there is a general readiness for primary nursing, then the ward or unit is at the 'get set' point. The next stage is the actual implementation, which on average seems to take about 18 months (this is a view derived from the experience of the contributors). For some it may be faster, for others, slower, depending upon the many variables:

Phase I The groundwork – perhaps years!

Phase II 6 months – preparing the staff. Reading about primary nursing; attending lectures; having meetings; planning the changes and how they will be managed; discussing primary nursing with others more experienced.

Phase III 6 months – the trial period. Putting the plans into action, all the time reviewing them; talking to each other; trying out the practice; identifying problems and overcoming them.

Phase IV 6 months of consolidation, rethinking and replanning. Refining the organisation of primary nursing and planning the moves towards perfection and identifying the limitations.

Planning the time phase, and making it realistic, is essential. Hoping for too much too soon can lead the staff to become dismayed and disillusioned. For example, leaping from task-centred care to primary nursing can be difficult for some; perhaps a transition phase, working at patient allocation first, can be helpful.

- *The choice of site.* It has been suggested that there is a time when a nursing unit becomes 'ripe' for primary nursing. This is rather difficult to define, but seems to be a combination of staff readiness, appropriate skill mix, staff willingness to try it, the supportive management climate and the knowledge and enthusiasm in sufficient key staff. Changing practice does not require everyone to be an enthusiastic innovator, but a small percentage of the workforce is sufficient to begin this transition. Some will lead, others will follow.

It seems that choosing the site, e.g. a ward or a team of community nurses where there is a willingness to learn and experiment, to act as a pilot scheme, is helpful. Other staff in other areas can learn from these schemes and perhaps reduce their own difficulties when they can learn from the experience of others. When one site is successful, then, rather like a germ, the idea can spread gradually from place to place, as Figure 2.2 illustrates.

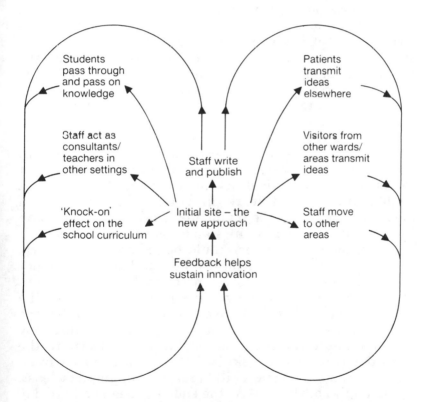

Fig. 2.2 Transmission of primary nursing beyond the pilot site (From Wright, 1986. Reproduced by kind permission of Edward Arnold)

This chapter has explained the concept of change in relation to primary nursing. There is no doubt that, as Machiavelli (1514) observed:

'There is nothing more difficult to handle, more doubtful of success, and more dangerous to carry through, than initiating changes in a state constitution. The innovator makes enemies of all those who progressed under the old order, and only lukewarm support is forthcoming from those who could prosper under the new'.

Perhaps the picture is not always as cynical and grim as Machiavelli would suggest. However, there can be little doubt that there are many health care settings where the mere suggestion of primary nursing would be greeted with disbelief, scorn or hostility. Faced in some places with a combination of inadequate numbers of nurses, unwilling staff and unsupportive managers or educators, then the prospect of change for primary nursing is indeed daunting. Sometimes presenting a good case can overcome the difficulties (e.g. tapping staff or management support by providing evidence of improved quality of care or better use of resources). At other times, nurses might move elsewhere if that is possible, to settings where their ideas will be received more positively. It is important, however, not to take on all the guilt if nursing does not always go as it might. Nurses often work in poor environments with inadequate resources, behaving in almost a 'heroic' fashion (Lanara, 1981) to maintain standards of care. When this happens, the guilty finger should be pointed quite clearly at the cause of the problem. If nurses fail, maybe it is not always because of weakness in themselves [as they are often made to feel (Salvage, 1985)]; rather, it is in the organisation and how it is governed and resourced that the problem lies. Nurses can help to change things by becoming more aware of the situation, by learning the skills of change agency (skills that can start to be learned on a good interpersonal skills programme) and, not least, by valuing what they do. At the end of a long and hard day (or night), it can seem hopeless to contemplate anything so seemingly remote as primary nursing. But there is a time and place for that. In the meantime, it is important to remember the good things that have been done, to contemplate the benefits, no matter how small, to patients and colleagues that each nurse offers each day – and to cherish them.

CHAPTER 3

The Nurse and the Patient in Primary Nursing

Just as the person who comes to see me needs me for help, I need him to express my ability to give help.

James Hillman
Insearch

Chapter 1 examined some of the central principles of primary nursing. These ideas now need to be developed a little further by looking not only at how the individual roles operate, but at some of the foundations required for the ethos of primary nursing to develop.

VALUING NURSING

Each member of the primary nursing team must value nursing and consider it important, worthwhile and therapeutic. At first sight, this may appear like an overly obvious statement to make, but in many respects nursing could be said to have got its values upside down. Trapped in a culture that espouses the rational, the scientific and the technological – dominated by the hospital-based medical model of care, wrapped up in the higher status associated with cure rather than care – so much of the heart of nursing has become devalued. Many thousands of nurses have come to see themselves in the 'narcissistic mirror offered by medicine' (Oakley, 1984).

Oakley argues that, in order to seek more autonomy, respect and recognition for what they do, nurses have become transfixed by the image in the mirror, not of themselves, but of medicine. In a still largely sexist society, male values predominate, and this is no less true than in male-dominated medicine. The masculine, scientific and rational mode is seen to have more value and status than the (feminine) caring and nurturing mode. Hence the (predominantly female) discipline of nursing has, to a large degree, pursued a false road. By allying itself to high-tech, acute, scientific medicine, it has hoped to gain from some of its status and power. Thus, areas associated with little medical intervention have traditionally had the lower status in nursing (and medicine), e.g. care of the elderly, the mentally handicapped and the mentally ill. The acute sector, associated with high medical intervention, focused on cure, has conversely been awarded higher status. Student nurses tended to gravitate to the latter field after qualification. Nursing has often been described in texts and discussed in classrooms as supportive to medical intervention. 'Basic' nursing is derided as simplistic or common sense – something that can be consigned to junior staff or untrained aides.

> I remember being in a room a few years ago discussing allocation of staff in the hospital. A very senior nurse in the acute area commented that all you need in 'geriatrics' is a weak brain and a strong back. I was furious. This was the 1980s. Still this attitude persisted amongst my senior nursing colleagues – 'geriatrics' was good enough for those who weren't too bright, who'd failed their finals, or, worse still, as punishment for those who'd transgressed in the acute sector.
>
> *Clinical nurse specialist*

Those who aspire to primary nursing recognise at the outset that:

There is no such thing as basic nursing

Those caring, nurturing, 'being with' skills are the very heart of nursing. Whether it be attending to patients' hygiene, teaching them to walk again, or comforting them when distressed, those activities are not 'basic' or 'menial' (though they are often derided as such); they are skills as valuable, complex and intricate as 'putting up the IVs' or 'giving the medicines as prescribed'.

Lanara (1981) suggests that the nature of so many of what have been put aside as 'basic' tasks are in fact nothing less than heroic acts. She writes:

'In nursing, there are no small and useless tasks. Every little thing counts and every moment weighs, since each is offered for the welfare of human beings. The nurse's work is a composite of significant moments. The high degree of responsibility, the intensity of attention, the alertness of the continuous watching of the critically ill patient, the unpredictability of emergencies, the feverish and laborious task: these are neither exceptions nor recurring cycles. They formulate the everyday rule of the nurse's load. But above and beyond the intensive stress which characterises every single nursing moment, what is known and incomprehensible to many is the heroism of the nurse's heart which, day by day, night by night, creates the unique meanings of nursing. Nursing constitutes an everyday synthesis of all the elements in spiritual grandeur, a grandeur which is inseparable from life's tragedy. Pain and suffering, the tragic element of human life in its greatest intensity and sharpness, constitute the matrix of nursing. And this cannot be transcended without heroism' (Lanara, 1981).

This is not to say that 'high-tech' intervention associated with curative medicine is not part of nursing, rather that it is peripheral to it. The nurse who does not value the heart of nursing, the expressive 'high-touch' role (in both the physical and psychological senses), has rejected nursing in favour of becoming some pseudo-technical assistant. Such a rejection demeans nursing, and turns the nurse into something else – a doctor's handmaiden? a technical

servant? a technician? Perhaps all these things and more –
anything, but not a nurse. Caring in nursing is healing, in
its own right – both separate from, and complementary to,
medicine. Nurses who have expanded their role by
enhancing, valuing and becoming expert in the 'being
with' skills have recognised its therapeutic nature. They
might still take on some technical medical task (i.e. use
instrumental skills), but only because it is an adjunct to
nursing (for example, the community nurse who carries out
intravenous injections as *part* of the total care given
during a visit) to promote a more holistic style of care.
However, this person is a very different nurse and holds a
very different set of values from the one who takes on such
tasks in order to gain some spurious status by seeming to
do 'clever' technical-medical functions. One of the
challenges for primary nursing is to combine the instrumental and expressive skills, yet retain the essential
nature of nursing, which is of value to both nurses and
patients.

We were at a conference discussing the content of the care plans. I
remember one nurse in the group being really dismissive of me. She didn't see
the point in what I regarded as important care; I mentioned things like
'staying with the patient when he is distressed', 'teaching him how to manage
the toilet' and 'getting another nurse to help me lift him'. 'These things are all
just common sense', she retorted, and then said: 'Anyway, don't you get
bored doing this sort of thing? I do ECGs, take blood, set up drips and things
like that. I get far more job satisfaction from this, have a good relationship
with my medical colleagues, and should be getting more pay.'

Clinical nurse specialist

Within the primary nursing system, nurses have a highly
developed set of values of what constitute nursing. They
identify where these roles interlock with other disciplines,
but in so doing have a clear image in their heads of what
nursing is. Primary nurses work *with* doctors and other
disciplines, not *for* them. They work *with* patients and the
families and not *at* or *to* them. Nurses immersed in primary
nursing have become 'conscious' about nursing. Woods

(1987), in explaining the black consciousness movement in South Africa, writes:

> 'The idea behind Black Consciousness was to break away almost entirely from past black attitudes . . . and to set a new style of self-reliance and dignity for blacks as a psychological attitude leading to new initiatives' (Woods, 1987).

There is a message here for nurses who embark along the road to primary nursing. If the word 'nursing' is transposed at appropriate points in the above quotation, then:

> 'The idea behind nursing consciousness was to break away almost entirely from past nursing attitudes . . . and to set a new style of self-reliance and dignity for nurses as a psychological attitude leading to new initiatives'.

The 'new initiative' of primary nursing requires more than a commitment to reorganise care; it requires nurses to develop and learn by their beliefs in the value of nursing.

Nursing as a Healing Act

Pearson (1988a) suggests that it is to nurses, more than any other group, that patients turn with the expectation that they will 'humanise' the system for them. When they do not, this contributes to the bulk of the complaints related to nursing which appear in, for example, the Health Service Ombudsman's reports (1986–1993). Nurses clearly have a responsibility to help people 'get better' – by contributing to various treatments, etc. – but they can also help people to 'feel better' (Kitson, 1988). Indeed, unless people 'feel better' – through sincere caring and comforting, the use of nursing expertise, interpersonal skills and so on – then it seems that the speed at which people 'get better' may be delayed. Even if the patient is dying, nursing can contribute to patients feeling better even when there is no possibility of recovery.

The success of nurses in this approach is based not so much on what nurses do, but how they do it. It is based less on technical, instrumental skills and more on the nature of the nurse–patient relationship. Patients appear to be very adept in identifying that certain something in a nurse which makes them feel comforted and reassured. In doing so, there is abundant evidence of a direct positive impact on the patient's health and well-being. Wounds are more likely to heal quickly, postoperative complications diminish, early discharge from hospital is more likely as is a general sense of well-being (and reduced death rates) when the influence of the nurse–patient relationship is recognised and applied effectively (Cassée, 1975; Wilson-Barnett and Carrigy, 1978; Wong, 1979; Pearson et al, 1992). Some of these features can be attributed to better communication skills among nurses, but there appear to be other factors which help to justify the argument that nursing itself is a therapeutic act (McMahon and Pearson, 1992). In other words, when nurses are able to demonstrate that they not only 'care for' people effectively (e.g. administer various treatments, attend to hygiene needs, assist with mobility and so on) but that they also 'care about' them – valuing, accepting, comforting the person as an individual – then the potential for nursing as a healing act in its own right is realised.

The loss of faith in medical intervention, coupled with perceptions that the existing health system does not 'care about' people enough, has led many to look elsewhere for help (Rankin-Box, 1993). There has been an enormous rise, for example, in the use of complementary therapies, partly because these seem to offer forms of treatment which are very focused on the individual with a high degree of personal attention. Paradoxically, many nurses also appear to be learning about these therapies themselves, in part because they seem to enhance the ability of nurses to demonstrate that they 'care about' their patients and promote healing and well-being (Sayre-Adams, 1993). Advertisements for courses and conferences in various therapies have proliferated in the nursing press, indicating that there is growing interest in these subjects. A special interest group in the RCN has one of the fastest expanding membership numbers in the organisation.

The attention paid to the complementary therapies may in part be symptomatic of the desire, by both nurses and patients, to experience a system of caring that is more humanised. Thus, implementing primary nursing in an organisational sense (i.e. allocating groups of nurses to patients) does not guarantee that the quality of care improves. Attention also has to be paid to the quality of the nurse–patient relationship. Applying the system of primary nursing, while it may put nurses in a good position to express and deliver nursing values, does not necessarily mean that they will do so. For some nurses, the shift of roles is easy and natural and enables them, with their existing knowledge and skill, to fulfil the needs of their patients and their own aspirations. Others need various forms of support and development to achieve this potential.

While primary nursing is a method of delivering care, it also has a philosophical dimension. It requires nurses to possess certain values about nursing and the contribution to the health and well-being of patients it can bring. These especially relate to the quality of the nurse–patient relationship and the qualities which the nurse brings to it. By combining the instrumental and expressive skills, the 'getting better' with the 'feeling better' acts, the 'caring for' with the 'caring about' approach, nurses bring the potent force of sincere, compassionate, creative concern for others into play. This is, of itself, therapeutic. Such a force represents a form of 'love' (Campbell, 1984; Chopra, 1989) where one human being is able to enter the world of others, to 'be with' them in times of need in ways which will comfort, help and heal.

'BEING WITH' THE PATIENT

Nurses involved in primary nursing work on the basis of a new relationship with patients. Wright (1986) and Pearson and Vaughan (1986) speak of 'partnership', and Campbell (1984) of 'companionship'. Both concepts appear to have very similar traits, and Campbell's definition appears to embody the main principles:

'A closeness which is not sexually stereotyped; it implies movement and change; it expresses mutuality; and it requires commitment, but within defined limits . . . companionship describes a closeness which is neither sexual union nor deep personal friendship. It is a bodily presence which accompanies the other for a while. The image of the journey springs to mind when we think of the companions.

Companionship often arises from a chance meeting and it is terminated when the joint purpose which keeps companions together no longer obtains. The good companion is someone who shares freely, but does not impose, allowing others to make their *own* journey' (Campbell, 1984).

Thus primary nurses work with patients, teaching, guiding and advising. They encourage patients to be involved in their own care, to make choices and give information so that the patient can make informed rational decisions. They share their knowledge and skills with the patient. They involve families, partners and other carers. Where other disciplines are involved, they work with them as part of a team to promote the patient's welfare. When the patients are unable or unwilling to make their wishes known, the primary nurse uses what knowledge is available of them, coupled with empathy skills, to act as advocate – upholding their wishes when they are unable to do so for themselves, advising in their best interests and being prepared to stand accountable for those decisions.

'Being with' is more than a mere bodily presence. It is, as Benner and Wrubel (1989) suggest, a complex act where nurses demonstrate their capacity to see the world from the patient's point of view, to 'bear witness' to their difficulties, hopes and histories, and like Campbell's (1984) 'companion' with a 'moderated' form of love, to offer help from a vast repertoire of healing, caring and comforting skills. Such a love, based on a genuine sincere concern for other human beings, transcends sexual interest or personal likes or dislikes or the traits in individual patients. It goes beyond these to see a fellow human being in need, and seeks to care with equal attentiveness, compassion and respect for all. This seems a great deal to ask of any nurse, but the evidence suggests that, often despite the difficulties of the system in which they work, thousands of nurses are struggling to achieve this goal every working day and night. 'Being with' patients is essential to the concept of primary nursing. Without it, primary nursing is just one more method of organising patient care. There is a good chance that improvements in care, making it more personal, will occur simply because the nurses' responsibilities are focused on a limited patient group. Patients will still be helped, probably more efficiently and effectively than in other systems. However, drawing on the dimension of 'moderated love' expands enormously the potential of the nurse–patient relationship into a therapeutic act.

With the above points in mind, perhaps Lathlean (1988) is correct when she asserts that 'Primary nursing can be more stressful than other ways of nursing, and therefore nurses need support to enable them to do the job effectively'. If primary nursing exhorts nurses to become involved with patients, then several profound issues arise.

The Value of Qualified Nursing

Unfortunately the 'caring about' dimension of nursing is often difficult to demonstrate and articulate. Lawler's research (1991) suggests that much of this work is 'invisible'. Thus, in the intensely cost-effective climate of modern health care, it can be very difficult for nurses to argue for appropriate levels of qualified staff. Where nursing is viewed by managers, and some nurses themselves, as basic tasks, then it is relatively easy to justify reducing the levels of qualified nurses on the assumption that more 'pairs of hands' (paid more cheaply) with a little training can do the work of nurses at less cost. If this scenario is followed to its logical conclusion, qualified nurses will be reduced to the role of supervisors of large groups of untrained or partially trained support workers. The added dimensions which qualified nursing can bring to the relationship with the patient will be lost.

The notion that nursing is somehow 'too expensive' and that nurses of the future, educated on P2000 courses, will be principally managers of others (mainly support workers) is being increasingly promulgated (Caines, 1990, 1993; Dyson, 1991). These views appear to misunderstand the purpose of P2000 (UKCC, 1986) which aims to produce 'questioning, creative practitioners'. An intent of P2000 is to equip more nurses with the 'being with' skills discussed earlier in this chapter. There seems little point in producing nurses of this calibre if they are to be used instead to manage the work of others. The views also appear to have fallen into the trap of misunderstanding or ignoring the complexity of nursing practice. 'Basic', 'simple' or 'menial' tasks are deemed worthy of delegation to others, their inherent value and intricacy in therapeutic nursing (and hence cost-effective care) are glided over. Nursing practice is a 'low level' activity – management and technology are viewed as tasks more worthy of nurses.

Once again, what these views have done is to turn the value of nursing on its head. The 'invisible' nature (Lawler, 1991) of much of nursing still leads many to underestimate its value and complexity. The evidence in favour of increasing rather than decreasing the number of qualified nurses in proportion to unqualified nurses is considerable. Numerous studies are now available pointing to the cost-effectiveness of qualified nursing (for example, Audit Commission, 1991; Buchan and Ball, 1991; Carr-Hill et al, 1992; North Western RHA, 1992; Pearson et al, 1992).

Many of these also indicate strong preferences for primary nursing as the organisational method of choice to enable nurses to work more efficiently and effectively. Short-term costs related to higher levels of qualified nurses in the skills mix ratio are outweighed by the longer-term benefits of the use of their therapeutic skills, not only in getting patients better, but helping them feel better too. Qualified nurses are more able to make decisions, and act without constant supervision – especially when placed in roles such as primary nursing which foster a higher degree of accountability and autonomy. In addition, primary nursing appears to bring cost savings in terms of recruitment, retention and effective performance of qualified staff (Chapter 6). As Payne (1991) suggests, 'There are cost benefits if you move the patient through the system more

efficiently. If you get it right in the first place, you don't need
to do the repairs. Money, time and frustration are wasted on
dealing with complaints, complications and so on'.

There appear to be many sound reasons for qualified
nurses working as primary nurses, not least the potential
cost benefit in the long term.

CAN AND DO ALL NURSES WISH TO BE PRIMARY NURSES?

The answer, quite simply, is no. Firstly, many nurses have
not accepted those values of nursing that underlie primary
nursing. This issue was covered in some depth earlier in
this chapter, and leaving this aside, there is the question of
how far nurses are able to be primary nurses. More
attention will be given to the educational preparation of
the primary nurse in Chapter 5. Certainly, the present
preparation of the nurse leaves much to be desired:

> 'It has been suggested that the roles of registered nurses and
> sisters are changed by primary nursing. Since we know that
> nurses are ill-prepared for their existing roles, they are even
> less likely to be prepared for new ones where, in the case of
> RGNs, greater autonomy and decision making are required. It
> could be argued that, when Project 2000 is implemented, this
> situation will be changed considerably, but it will be a long
> time before the full effects are felt. Post-basic and continuing
> educational opportunities vary tremendously across the
> country, and professional development schemes for registered
> nurses are only beginning to be offered by health authorities'
> (Lathlean, 1988).

Benner (1984) further argues that what constitutes the
real nature of nursing is often not taught or valued, and
that producing the 'professional' nurse can take many
years, certainly more than a basic 3-year programme. A
precursor to primary nursing must therefore be the
preparation of the nurses. As was suggested in Chapter 2,
this might take at least 6 months of further education of
the staff, before primary nursing is implemented (more
details on suggested content of such preparation are
included in Chapter 5). Furthermore it is not just a

question of preparation beforehand, but it should be part of a *nursing lifetime* of continuing education and development.

A PRIMARY NURSING CULTURE

Nurses, Menzies (1961) argued, are ill-equipped to cope with the anxiety of the fraught world of nursing and need task allocation to shield them from involvement with the patient. If it is now suggested that nurses become involved, along the lines described by Campbell (1984) as 'companions' or 'partners', how can this challenge be met? If the crutches of task allocation are pulled away, what is needed to replace them so that the nurse does not collapse under the weight of anxiety and stress in her role?

Part of the answer is to equip the nurse with the 'survival skills' (see Chapter 5) that are needed, including assertiveness and self-awareness. Another part is to develop the climate in which primary nursing and the nurses involved in it can be fostered and nourished. A nursing culture can be produced where the hallmarks are as follows:

- A non-hierarchical, team approach to care.
- Managers and educators are supportive, 'walk the patch', listen to staff views, give praise to reinforce the staff, provide opportunities for further development and support innovation.
- A spirit exists in the team that embodies a 'we are all in this together' approach. Nurses in the team feel free to ask questions and seek advice and support from colleagues, and are not belittled when they do.
- Change, innovation, research and learning are considered to be just as important as getting through the work.
- There is an openness, a willingness to share experiences and a flexibility in relationships with colleagues, patients, relatives and others.
- The philosophy of the unit is shared by all; goals and objectives and decisions are jointly agreed.

- The staff place a high value on nursing, and upon holistic and individualised approaches to care.
- Routines and rituals are minimised; the climate supports flexibility in nurse–patient activities.

Good teamwork is as essential to managing change as it is to primary nursing. A climate of openness and honesty helps to reassure staff, allay anxiety and minimise resistance. It also fosters the shared sense of common purpose which is essential to high quality patient care. The staff of the Tameside unit found that Manthey's words (1988b) succinctly summarised their feelings (Figure 3.1).

It could be argued that factors such as these should be the norm in any nursing setting. Unfortunately, many nurses do not experience such benefits (Price Waterhouse, 1988; Buchan and Seccombe, 1991). A primary nursing culture is essential to the creation and maintenance of primary nursing and to the welfare of both patients and staff involved in it.

> I remember as a student being 'ticked off' for sitting talking with a patient. 'Haven't you anything to do?', I was asked. It's not like that here. I have my patients. If talking with them is part of their needs, then I get on with it. The team here know what nursing is. They've got their priorities right.
>
> *Primary nurse*

AUTONOMY AND ACCOUNTABILITY

Making decisions about care, being free to carry them out, and accepting responsibility for the effects underpin the role of the primary nurse. However, as Bergman (1981) points out, professional freedom to this degree means that nurses must have the ability to make such decisions and to take on such responsibility as well as having the authority to pursue them. The bureaucratic nature of much of health care and the status of nursing within it leaves nurses in a very hazy position.

Dimond (1988), as a barrister with a particular interest and expertise in nursing issues, has argued that, in law,

The Nursing Development Unit

THE TEAM –
A COMMITMENT TO EACH OTHER

$\boxed{A}$s your colleague in a team dedicated to providing excellent nursing care to our patients, I commit myself to the following:

- I will accept responsibility for establishing and maintaining healthy interpersonal relationships with you and every member of the staff. I will talk to you promptly if I am having a problem with you. The only time I will discuss it with another person is when I need advice or help in deciding how to talk with you properly.

- I will establish and maintain a relationship of trust with you and every member of the staff. My relationships with each of you will be equally respectful, regardless of job titles or levels of educational preparation.

- I will not engage in the "3 B's" (bickering, backbiting and bitching) and will ask you not to as well.

- I will not complain about another team member, and ask you not to as well. If I hear you doing so I will ask you to talk to that person.

- I will accept you as you are today, forgiving past problems and ask you to do the same.

- I will be committed to finding solutions to problems, rather than complaining about them or blaming someone for them, and ask you to do the same.

- I will affirm your contribution to quality patient care.

- I will remember that neither of us is perfect, and that human errors are opportunities, not for shame or guilt but for forgiveness and growth.

(based on an original work by Marie Manthey, (1988))

Caring for the Elderly

Fig. 3.1 Nursing team commitment poster

nursing care essentially remains within the domain of the doctor. Recent trends, however, have been pushing the nurse further and further along the road to professional autonomy and accountability. The Code of Professional Conduct and Project 2000 (UKCC, 1983 and 1986 respectively) envisage a nurse who is directly accountable to the patient. Subsequent updating papers (UKCC, 1992a, b) place nurses quite clearly as individually accountable to patients for their actions, regardless of the organisational methods they use.

The limits to autonomy and accountability are somewhat hazy for both legal and practical reasons. Autonomy in primary nursing, for example, is unlikely to be achievable in every sense (control over decisions and actions) since nurses often work in teams, with responsibilities to each other and more senior nurses and managers. Many aspects of care are often compromised by financial restrictions, organisational rules and legal responsibilities to patients and doctors. Some organisations are quite explicit about what nurses can and cannot do, including speaking out about internal problems to other individuals, the media and so on (Hancock, 1991b).

Precedents set by legal proceedings, Acts of Parliament and guidelines laid down by professional bodies are providing the frameworks for nursing autonomy. It will be different for nursing, as it is with each other profession. Autonomy in primary nursing is unlikely to come to mean complete and unbridled freedom of action (Johns, 1990). It seems more likely that it relates to a degree of freedom of decision-making and delivery of patient care based on the nurse's own knowledge and skills, and for a given caseload of patients and within the framework of a clearly identified role. The autonomy to practise at this level will be bounded and muddied by contracts with employers, the collective responsibilities negotiated in the team and the limits to the power over resources and the knowledge and skills which nurses possess.

There can be little doubt that nurses who assert professional autonomy and choose to accept their accountability are skating on the thin ice at the outer edges of the profession. Some nurses (for example, those who raised objections to electroconvulsive therapy) have found this to their cost.

In practice, the legal position is very unclear and often ill-considered by nurses. At the same time, fears over litigation are often thrown up as an excuse for not changing, or for not trying anything new. Primary nursing is about putting into action what is in effect a worldwide nursing phenomenon – the desire for professional self-determination. It is certain that the legal framework in which this is carried out needs to be clarified to remove the uncertainty from nurses and the attendant sense of risk.

While many fears over 'What happens if . . .?' may surface in nurses from time to time, such risks need to be set in perspective. The reality is that most nurses work well in team relationships with colleagues, and problems that get to the point of litigation are relatively minimal. This is not to underestimate the importance of the issue, rather to set it more realistically in context.

We decided to press on with our plans to let the patients have access to their nursing plans. We agreed as a team and kept other colleagues, including the doctors, informed. It's worked well, but part of the reason seems to be us, the way we work together here. I know someone who tried the same idea in another place, and it was squashed before it even got off the ground. He was given all kinds of legal reasons why it wouldn't work, and one doctor refused permission anyway. So, it never happened – 'too dangerous', he was told. I ask you, if nurses worked on that basis all the time, you'd never get past your front door! I often think that the relationship you build up with colleagues, so that you are trusted and respected, is as important as any legal framework. I know what I am and how to do it, and am quite prepared to stand up and be counted if I drop a clanger! I do not need someone else to *permit* me to decide what nursing is, though I understand in law that's strictly speaking the doctor's prerogative. Well, laws change, customs and practice change. I'd rather we led the way on this than sat forever under the doctor's coat-tails or hid behind the hospital procedure book! We work well here, we've a collegial relationship that works, and it works because we each know where the other stands, and what each other's jobs are.

Senior primary nurse/ward sister

Nurses who set out primary nursing are, to some degree, pursuing a professional adventure. If they take on the perceptions of autonomy to practise and accountability to the patient, they must also take on board the implications that go with them. While some nurses may feel uncertain about autonomy and accountability aspects, it may be argued that nurses within the primary nursing system may feel more secure, not less so. The clarification of roles and responsibilities makes it easier to identify who should be dealing with a problem and who is responsible for the actions taken. Such responsibilities appear to be less stressful than working in teams, where the boundaries are unclear. Not only are there greater freedoms in decision-making about nursing practice, there are also greater responsibilities (of keeping up to date, of maintaining high standards, of practising on the basis of sound knowledge, of being prepared to be accountable, and so on) which go with them.

THE ROLES

This chapter concludes with a brief outline of the principal roles in primary nursing and how they work with patients (and others) in the revised way discussed above. It is essential that these rules are clarified within the team/with managers in order to minimise the risks of confusion over autonomy and accountability mentioned above. Throughout the literature on primary nursing, there are three key roles envisaged: primary nurse, associate nurse and care assistant. How far each of these roles fits with the principal existing clinical jobs in the UK, e.g. sister/charge nurse/staff nurse/enrolled nurse/nursing auxiliary/assistant, will be discussed in more detail in Chapter 4.

The Primary Nurse

The primary nurse is seen as a registered (first level) nurse, having undertaken at least a 3-year programme of education. This is the key role responsible for assessing, planning, implementing and evaluating the care of the patient from admission through to discharge or transfer. This nurse is accountable for the care that is prescribed and given, and may have added responsibilities in teaching, researching and managing others in the nursing team involved in the patient's care. The primary nurse co-ordinates the patient's nursing care, as well as liaising with other members of the multidisciplinary team to ensure that it is comprehensive. This includes working with relatives, visitors and others. The primary nurse might be seen as sitting at the centre of the web of care with the patient, working as a partner and companion in care, and pulling together all the many strands involved in his health and well-being. The primary nurse is knowledgeable and autonomous, basing practice on sound rationale, yet seeking help, advice and further self-development to ensure that the practice is up to date. The primary nurse works with colleagues, using a nursing model to generate nursing practice, and participates in the evaluation of care in the wider sphere, for example in quality assurance programmes to ensure that the delivery of care is of the highest quality.

The primary nurse prepares the patient for discharge and joins in the multidisciplinary team decision on this issue. In some units, the primary nurse may also have designated 'nursing beds' where medical intervention is relatively small. The primary nurse may control the admission and discharge of patients in these beds. Having nursing beds, however, is not essential to primary nursing.

The Associate Nurse

This nurse need not necessarily be a registered nurse (although the primary nurse can 'act across' for a colleague's patients and care for them as an associate nurse in his/her absence). The associate nurse cares for the patient in the absence of the primary nurse, and may adjust the care as necessary. Major changes are carried out in consultation with the primary nurse. In some settings, this may mean that the primary nurse may work 'on call' or suggest being contacted even when off duty if a particular issue of importance crops up. In practice, these should only be on rare occasions. Where the associate nurse is not a registered nurse, then the primary or another registered (primary) nurse must be available to monitor the patient's care and offer help and guidance if needed. Continuity of care is essential and must be backed up by written care plans and effective verbal reporting methods. The associate nurse works very closely with the primary nurse to co-ordinate the patient's care and contribute to a rich information exchange, so that all facets of the patient's care can be constantly monitored and evaluated.

If the primary nurse delegates care to an unqualified nurse, then accountability for that care remains with the primary nurse. The primary nurse is responsible for ensuring that the person taking over aspects of care in his or her absence is competent to do so. The associate nurse is not necessarily a more 'junior' nurse. Often it can be a role used by ward sisters/charge nurses or nurse specialists who may take temporary responsibility for a caseload of patients but who, for other reasons, are not able to act as primary nurses (see Chapter 4).

In the absence of the primary nurse, the qualified associate nurse remains accountable in his or her own right and can adjust the plan of care accordingly. Primary nursing does not mean that the associate nurse must not do anything unless the primary nurse has made the decision.

The Care Assistant

These assistants help the primary nurses and associate nurses by carrying out the non-nursing duties essential to the order of a unit. They may assist the primary and associate nurses in the giving of care (e.g. helping them to bath a patient or helping with lifting or exercises). They may help, for example, with the preparation and serving of meals, with bed-making and with the general orderliness and upkeep of the ward. Although not a trained nurse, the care assistant is included with others as part of the nursing team and is expected to contribute to decisions about the unit as well as to offer observations on patients and their progress in the overall evaluation of the patient's care.

Many care assistants have undertaken training for their role, including the recently developed National Vocational Qualification (NVQ) programme for support workers. Clearly, carers with these aspects of training cannot be primary nurses or associate nurses, because they are not by definition nurses on the register held by the professional body. In some settings, support workers (depending on their level of training) are involved as associate carers, working under the supervision of a qualified nurse. If the primary nurse is absent, another qualified nurse should be available to provide the necessary supervision. Where this is not so, the qualified nurse needs to be satisfied that the assistant is competent to carry out any care delegated, and the assistant remains responsible to the primary nurse. The primary nurse remains accountable overall for the care given.

Although different roles have been developed in the primary nursing system, it is important to stress that this does not remove the need to work as a team. The roles in primary nursing are not about status and seniority, but describe the *function* which nurses and others undertake within their roles. Thus the primary nurse is not necessarily the most 'senior' in the team, and the associate nurse not the most 'junior'. Primary nursing is not concerned with creating new hierarchies to replace old ones, but with establishing clearer lines of responsibility and accountability to each other and to patients.

The primary nurse is responsible for making a plan of care for each patient in our group, and my job is to work with these patients and nurse for the whole of my shift, helping to give the care planned for them.

I am always fully informed of their condition. I get a full verbal report and can have an input to their care planning, e.g. reporting on bowel movements or incontinence episodes, etc. I can contribute to the hand-over report for these patients and tell the staff about any changes I've

continued next page

continued

observed. This information is always listened to, and is of value to trained staff in planning the nursing care. We work closely as a team and have regular meetings for discussions, and all staff participate. I sit in on case conferences held for the patient and am made to feel my judgment is trusted and valued.

I assist my nurse with patient care – washing, dressing, toiletting, etc., as well as seeing to the general orderliness of the ward. By working as a member of a small team looking after a small group of patients, I am left time to do other activities with them – letter writing, crossword puzzles or hairstyling – or simply just talking with and listening to them.

Primary nursing has meant that I now have the time and the opportunity to build up a good and sometimes quite close relationship with the patients. I find it more rewarding to be with both patients and staff in this way.

The care assistant has a significant role to play in supporting primary nursing. He or she needs to feel fully involved as part of the team, and should also be given opportunities for education and personal development to help them fulfil it to the maximum.

Care assistant

The above provides a general outline of the main roles, and clearly there is a need for co-ordination of these activities. The role of the ward sister/charge nurse remains 'key' (Pembrey, 1980) in this respect. More details of these organisational matters are discussed in Chapter 4.

SUMMARY

Nursing is a healing presence with patients, and this chapter has sought to develop further areas on how primary nursing can enhance that presence as well as look at some of the concerns for the nurses and patients involved. This type of involvement requires considerable skill and commitment, and yet more, for it is not too grand a word to use to suggest that it takes 'love', a 'moderated love' (Campbell, 1984) that helps both nurse and patient to find their way through the complexity of their relationship and dependence on each other. This love requires respect for the individual on the part of the nurse, a genuine desire to help another human being in what might, at the very least, be difficult and distressing times. Nurses are frequently called upon to transmit this love, often against great odds of poor staffing levels and resources. When they fail to do so, they can feel bad about themselves, even though their lack of preparedness, of support, of resources, is the real root of the problem. Nurses involved in primary nursing are tapping that love in the often heroic effort to do what is best for the patient. It is a love which rests on the recognition of the value of nursing and of the nurse.

Primary nursing thus demands much of its nurses, but it has the potential to give so much to them and their patients in return. Many contentious issues and problems have so far been raised, and in the next chapter we will look at how some of these can be resolved.

CHAPTER 4

Organisational Matters

People will tell you where they've gone,
They'll tell you where to go
But till you get there yourself, you never really know

Joni Mitchell (1976)
Amelia
From the album 'Hejira' on Asylum Records

Every setting, every nurse, is unique. Thus, all the contributors to this text are wary of being prescriptive. From the experience of dealing with the thousands of visitors who have been to Tameside's Nursing Development Unit, the kind of questions and concerns raised by nurses tend to be very similar. Often what nurses seek is a magic box, filled with all the right answers: 'Give me your box that I may go away and do likewise!'

The principles of primary nursing are universal but the application is open to many options. Flexibility is the key. Anything that nurses do to make care more personal, often in very difficult circumstances, needs to be valued and cherished, whether it is full-blown primary nursing or not. Indeed there are many simple acts – a shift in the ward routine here, an adjustment to the usual ritual there – that nurses can accomplish without a great deal of effort or resources to improve the lot of both patients and nurses. Sometimes it is difficult to judge which comes first – a climate of hope and innovation from which primary nursing is but a natural step, or primary nursing (or just thinking about it) which sets the ball of innovative practice rolling.

Whichever is the case (and it is probably a combination of both), experience has confirmed what has been suggested in the previous chapters – there comes a time. It is difficult to describe or measure. It is intangible, qualitative and intuitive, but a time comes when a place is ripe for primary nursing – that peculiar combination of circumstances of people and the place that transforms the situation beyond 'on your marks' to 'get set, then go'.

The rest of this chapter is therefore devoted not only to answering some of the very common questions that arise when nurses embark on primary nursing, but also to dealing with the problems and questions that arise once the process is under way. The questions here deal principally with the 'doing' of primary nursing and are set in no particular order of priority.

1. What Happens to the Role of the Ward Sister/ Charge Nurse?

In short it undergoes a radical transformation from the traditional role, i.e that of total controller of the nursing team and their actions. Primary nursing is about the unleashing of the individual autonomy and accountability of each primary nurse. It is incompatible with rigid, autocratic, hierarchical forms of nursing, whether in hospital or the community.

The sister or charge nurse is still the key figure, but in different ways. Primary nursing will not work unless he or she lets it. The role changes dramatically, new roles are taken on and some old ones discarded.

Senior primary nurse/charge nurse

If each primary nurse is to practise with the maximum degree of autonomy, the role of the ward sister remains 'key' (Pembrey, 1980) to the success. However, primary nursing is not a charter for anarchy. Nurses operate on very different levels of experience and knowledge of nursing (Benner, 1984), and it is the ward sister or charge nurse who has developed to the level of expert who acts as the support to colleagues. Some of these nurses will have achieved this level of expertise and can then be given full rein for their autonomy, the sister/charge nurse acting as the support person to enable them to get on with the job. For others, a higher degree of monitoring and supervision may be needed to ensure that all clinical decisions are accurate and safe. This can produce a dilemma for the clinical team and there is a danger here of giving conflicting signals (on the one hand letting go, on the other checking up on what nurses do). Ultimately, how well this works depends upon the strength of the team, the nature of the collegial relationship and the degree of trust embodied between colleagues. It is these that ensure that the managerial powers of the sister/charge nurse are used and interpreted in the team not as, 'I'm in charge and I'm watching what you're doing because I'm unsure of you or you're not experienced enough', but as, 'Because of my experience and the authority I've been given, I'm here to help you, support you and guide you in your practice so that both you and the patient don't come to harm'.

The sister or charge nurse, whether in hospital or community, as the overall leader of the team has a crucial role to play as 'clinical leader' – the clinical expert who guides and coaches the team, using a variety of clinical supervision techniques (Butterworth and Faugier, 1992). Supervision of this type has to do less with hierarchical control of staff based on the use of power and authority, and more with monitoring, supporting and developing the clinical competence and expertise of the nursing team. The use of clinical supervision has recently been strongly advocated in the 'Vision for Nursing' targets (NHSME, 1993).

The difference in style is distinct, but subtle, and there is no underestimating the interpersonal skills this key person must have to do it effectively. Primary nursing, while fostering autonomy, is not an unbridled licence for all nurses to act without question or supervision. Not all nurses have achieved the level of expert; not all have total awareness of the limitations to their knowledge and skill. The working relationship with the team leader – the sister/charge nurse – will vary with each member of that team according to their unique qualities. Encouraging primary nurses towards autonomy does not mean that the team leader abrogates his or her role as professional adviser, monitor and co-ordinator of care (Figure 4.1).

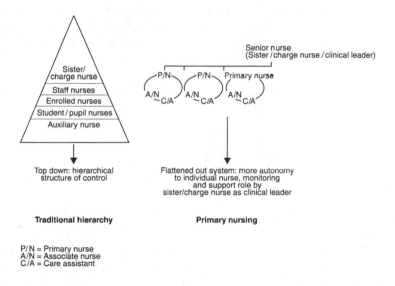

Fig. 4.1 The changed nature of the team relationship in primary nursing (After Sparrow, 1986)

I have to be sure of myself as a clinical practitioner and manager to take on the role. My ward does not lend itself to my being a primary nurse, I leave that to the others. I have chosen to work as an associate nurse. I see myself as the lynch-pin on the ward, yet at the same time I have to be able to

continued next page

continued

devolve responsibility and decision making. I have to let them get on with it yet be there to support them and make sure that all decisions and actions are the right ones. It doesn't mean I'm breathing down their necks all the time — we wouldn't have primary nursing if that were the case. It's more subtle than that, difficult to explain, but you know when it's working. I think in part, you get there when the staff see you as a sort of nursing consultant. You know you're on the right track when their self-awareness (in part developed by you) is such that they approach *you* for help because they know they are at the limits of their knowledge or skill.

Senior primary nurse/charge nurse

The effects of this shift of role for the 'captain of the team' vary according to the current style the sister/charge nurse already used. In some it is a natural development; for others it can be a radical shift, an almost terrifying experience.

I found that I needed peer support too. I have to support everybody else, but what about me! The support of management and colleagues is crucial. You go through all kinds of feelings, because you're brought up to be in control, to be 'in charge'. You feel uncomfortable at first, a bit insecure, and have to be wary of rushing to the defences and getting authoritarian again. It just takes time, you work through it.

Senior primary nurse/ward sister

The role of the ward sister/charge nurse, therefore, undergoes considerable changes with primary nursing. From being the 'head of the ward, fount of all knowledge, decisions not be questioned' figure, he or she becomes the 'navigator' of the ward or unit, giving it direction and a sense of cohesion, and helping to set the vision for nursing which the whole team pursue. The roles of counsellor, facilitator, supporter, teacher and researcher are enhanced (roles which the sister/charge nurse is expected to fulfil anyway) and come more to the fore. The sister/charge nurse may be the principal change agent (Chapter 2) helping to take forward the implementation of primary nursing. Indeed, freed of 'total control', the sister/charge nurse has the time to give to these functions, and to be a more effective manager and user of the resources of the unit.

> I had to become a counsellor, teacher, guide all in one. I saw it as my job to create the climate where we could all grow as a team, express views and seek advice freely without anxiety or fear of recrimination. We have regular meetings – planned and ad hoc, social gatherings, and working groups looking into certain topics. I delegated all kinds of things to the others, one primary nurse looking after the off-duty, another monitoring the holidays, someone else to keep an eye on the stocks and stores. We set up a quality circle. Individual nurses were designated as 'information seekers' when a topic or problem came up, to report back to the whole team on their findings; others meanwhile were encouraged to become the ward 'mini' specialist, for example one for continence advice, another for pressure area care. All these ideas were really to get over to the team that responsibilities were devolved.
>
> *Senior primary nurse/charge nurse*

The sister/charge nurse has a key role to play too, in developing both self and colleagues, keeping up to date by reading journals, attending courses and conferences, and so on, as an inherent part of primary nursing (as it should be in all aspects of nursing!). The team leader has the task of fostering the development not only of him/herself, but also of colleagues in the team. Without a sense of continuous learning and development, primary nursing can shrivel up.

2.   Can the Sister/Charge Nurse be a Primary Nurse?

Yes, in both hospital and community settings. In the community, where the nurse works on a one-to-one basis with patients and families, this is relatively straightforward. (Indeed, some community nurses would agree that they have always been primary nurses.) In hospitals or nursing homes dealing with larger groups of staff, then many alternatives are available depending on the individual characteristics (patient dependency, skill mix, staffing levels, etc.) of each setting, for example:

• Sister/charge nurse takes full caseload of patients (equal to other primary nursing colleagues).
• Takes reduced caseload as primary nurse while focusing on other duties.
• Does not act as primary nurse but as an associate nurse to a specific primary nurse.
• Acts neither as associate nor primary nurse, but remains free to deal with other activities, or 'floats', and takes over as associate or primary nurse (e.g. during sickness or absence of associate nurse or primary nurse).

Lathlean (1988) is of the view that:

'The sister, unless acting as a primary nurse, does not prescribe or actually give care. She acts as the co-ordinator of nursing staff, a resource and information provider and, importantly support giver – a role which differs greatly from that of the traditional sister.

In practice, the person occupying this role may be given an alternative title to highlight the differences. Some health authorities are developing senior roles, known as senior sisters, where the occupant is responsible for the management of a ward's nursing budget, decisions about skill mix of nursing staff and the provision of expert advice, without day-to-day accountability for the care of individual patients'.

Whichever of the above, or combination of them, is chosen must depend on a flexible approach based on the qualities of the particular unit. Depending on the level of commitment as primary nurse, the sister/charge nurse can act as overall co-ordinator of the ward. In other instances, the primary nurses may share this load and rotate ward co-ordinating functions amongst themselves. Whichever is the case, it is important that the sister or charge nurse remains a clinician in order to be an effective role model, whether it be as primary nurse or associate nurse.

3. Who Is the Primary Nurse?

There is general agreement that the primary nurse must be a first level registered nurse, as has been suggested earlier. This is based on a combination of factors (preparation during training, legal responsibilities, codes of conduct, etc.). The primary nurse must be a competent practitioner, able to assess, plan, deliver and evaluate care for a given caseload of patients. The primary nurse is a direct care giver, though may not necessarily be giving all of it. Some may be delegated to others in the team who are not nurses, or handed over to associate nurses when the primary nurse is absent. However, as Benner (1984) has noted, there can be a great variation in expertise between individual nurses, and Manthey (1970) notes how 'Experience as well as education must be taken into account when assessing an individual nurse's level of expertise in caring for various levels of patients'. It may well be that in terms of knowledge, skill and experience, an individual enrolled nurse might be better equipped to deliver a patient's care than a newly qualified RGN. The position of the enrolled nurse will be dealt with below. The primary nurse, meanwhile, requires a rolling programme of support and professional development to achieve the level of expert in care. It must run in parallel with the nurse's gradual development in practice, so that, over time, the primary nurse gradually becomes an expert autonomous practitioner.

4. What about the Enrolled Nurse?

Having two levels of qualified nurse in British nursing has produced many problems, and primary nursing forces a confrontation with some of these issues. In principle, the primary nurse is a first level registered nurse. Yet many settings have a higher dependency on enrolled nurses (and would have difficulty in recruiting otherwise). Where the enrolled nurse works as a primary nurse, then a number of factors need to be considered:

- The enrolled nurse him/herself, without pressure, agrees with being a primary nurse, and this is done on the basis of informed consent, i.e. he/she has been fully informed about primary nursing, in particular the knowledge and skills needed and the relationship to accountability, and is therefore still willing to take on the role.
- The enrolled nurse has been adequately prepared for the role (Smith and Atkinson (1992) suggest a special course for this).
- The unit's staff and management are in agreement on the issue, and this agreement is fully documented.

> It needs to be mentioned that this issue must be handled delicately if the enrolled nurse is not to feel that she is not trusted. It requires a degree of understanding and mutual support amongst the staff and a recognition that these precautions are taken, not because 'we don't trust the SEN' but because we need to ensure that she is adequately supported and covered in the unlikely event of something going wrong.
>
> *Primary nurse*

It has been argued that when the enrolled nurse takes on the role, the legal framework is somewhat doubtful. It is also worth noting that if the enrolled nurse is skilled enough to act as a primary nurse, then he/she should be fully educated (e.g. offered a conversion course) and paid as such.

There is no doubting the very real dilemma surrounding the role of the enrolled nurse (EN) in primary nursing, particularly in settings where they are a large part of the nursing workforce. Some of these aspects therefore need also to be considered:

- The primary nurse role (the word 'primary' has a ring of higher status or importance about it) should not be put forward as more important than other roles. The primary nurse does not function without the associate nurse and vice versa.

When we explained to the ENs what primary nursing was all about, a lot of rethinking went on. It is absolutely essential to ensure that the associate nurse role (which seemed to us to be a more appropriate role for the EN) is *valued*. I can't stress this enough. It's an important part of the whole approach, so you can't afford to have people feeling they occupy some second rate role. Taking this approach, most of our SENs have been happy in this capacity.

Nurse manager

Valuing the role of the associate nurse is a vital step in removing problems over status or of feeling devalued. This must happen within the whole team in order to develop the right niche for the enrolled nurse who chooses not to be a primary nurse.

• A strategy (and it may well be a long-term one) might need to be developed for revising the skill mix in a unit (see Chapter 6), gradually helping more enrolled nurses to undertake conversion courses (if they wish to do so) and steadily increasing the proportion of first level registered nurses to other grades of staff.

There tend to be conflicting issues in nursing in relation to status and qualification. As has been suggested earlier, the roles in primary nursing describe *function*, not *status*. If the enrolled nurse in the team is feeling devalued, or receives signals from others that they regard themselves 'as more important', then this is an important problem to be dealt with. It says little about primary nursing and more about problems within the team, and perhaps some team building exercises are necessary. A strong team spirit of positive collegial relationships is needed, in which all roles are valued as essential to primary nursing (McMahon, 1990a; Mead, 1990a).

It must also be remembered that qualifications alone will not determine who should or should not be a primary nurse. The determining factor is one of *competence*, and all nurses are bound by their own code of conduct not to undertake anything with patients for which they do not feel competent.

Enrolled nurses, for example, are trained to *assist* in the assessing, planning, giving and evaluating of care. The primary nurse has to be able to carry these out independently. However, the qualification only determines skills at the point at which they qualify, and does not take account of subsequent development and experience. The latter may be judged in ways other than formal qualification (e.g. peer review, appraisal) and also requires the nurse to be satisfied him/herself of being competent to practise in the role. This includes being able to demonstrate the necessary knowledge base and skills to be able to function as a primary nurse. Enrolled nurses need to bear these factors in mind when decisions are made about who shall and shall not be a primary nurse. It is important to examine and work in the role most appropriate to the level of competence. It is also important to ensure that they are not exploited as cheap labour, and given the responsibility of being a primary nurse without the appropriate level of pay, as in the UK, according to the clinical grading criteria. It is quite clear from the latter that Scale E is the minimum appropriate for someone working as a primary nurse.

5.   What about Staffing Levels and Skill Mixes?

According to Watson (1978) these must be *adequate* and *consistent*. She recommends the following:

Patients per primary nurse	Type of care
2	Critical care unit
5	Acute
7	Long term

Thus on a ward of 25 acutely ill patients, there would need to be at least 5 RGNs (full time) acting as primary nurses, with sufficient numbers of associate nurses (Watson argues for 2·5 per primary nurse) and care assistants to continue the care in the absence of the primary nurse. In addition to the number of staff, getting the skill mix right can be a difficult issue and may be the subject of longer term planning before primary nursing begins (see Chapter 2). The problems here can be aggravated by local recruitment difficulties, the popularity/unpopularity of the specialty, and so on. However, the experience of some units (Pearson, 1988a; Purdy et al, 1988) suggests that moves towards primary nursing can enhance staff recruitment so that the desired skill mix can be achieved. This appears to support the findings of other research (McClure et al, 1983; Price Waterhouse, 1988) that nurses are attracted to areas in which they feel they can practise nursing with greater autonomy and freedom.

We wanted to do primary nursing years ago, but with 80% of the workforce untrained it seemed a pipe-dream. Over the years we've adjusted the mix as people have left – now we have 65% trained staff, and the pipe-dream can be a reality.

Consultant nurse and nurse manager

There is still much debate relating to appropriate skill mix of nurses in relation to patient dependency, partly because so much of nursing is difficult to measure, as is the quality of care delivered. Watson's paper, cited above, must be taken as very generalised figures that can be used as a basis for agreeing staffing levels and mixes. In some units (e.g. intensive care or the critically ill patient on the general ward), a one-to-one relationship may be necessary. Other writers have indicated greater variations in these figures [up to 11 or 12 patients per primary nurse in continuing care settings (Hegyvary, 1982; Tutton, 1986)].

On our unit, we found that five or six patients per primary nurse is a comfortable ratio, and with very little variation between the acute and continuing care wards. That's not to say that the primary nurse looks after her patients and no others. Sometimes the primary nurse can act as an associate nurse for another primary nurse. The ward sister only takes a caseload of one or two patients, and the rest of the back-up team make up the total number of staff on the ward.

Primary nurse

The total number of staff on the ward must reflect the individual characteristics of the setting, and as yet no completely reliable tools for making calculations have emerged.

> The skill mix change was most important to us; what we found was that quality, not quantity, matters. There are fewer 'bodies' on the ward, in terms of the total number of staff, but practice is much more autonomous, i.e. I wouldn't have to waste my time supervising numbers of untrained staff.
>
> *Primary nurse*

As MacGuire (1988) succinctly points out: 'The exact values of staff at different levels may be less important largely because of the great variability on a day-to-day basis at ward level. What does matter is that we look at what is happening at the ward level and make the most of the skills and abilities which are there'.

The numbers of patients that each primary nurse will accept on his or her caseload will depend upon several variables including:

• the skills and experience of the individual nurse and the team members;
• the needs/dependency level of the patients;
• the environment/geography of the clinical area.

Thus, an experienced primary nurse may be able to manage the care of a larger caseload than a less experienced one. A very ill patient may require the full attention of one nurse. A nurse caring for patients located over a wide area of a ward or community will be able to care for fewer patients than if they were grouped closely together.

It may well be that even within one area, different nurses will have different sizes of caseload. One primary nurse on a ward may be entirely committed to one very ill patient, while another in the same ward may have a larger number, because the patients may be less dependent. To help to make decisions in this area, many groups of nurses have developed simple dependency scoring systems to ensure that they do not overload themselves and to help to spread the workload fairly.

6. How Are Patients Allocated to Nurses?

In some instances, allocation of patients is made by the most senior nurse (head nurse or ward sister/charge nurse), otherwise by mutual agreement of the primary nurses. The choice should be made by the staff on site. Varying lengths of stay of patients, staffing levels and skill mixes may mean that the number of patients per primary nurse may vary even within one unit. Assessment on the basis of the scope of patients' needs, not just physical status, is the determining factor. In addition, the patient may wish to have a say in who his or her primary nurse might be (see question 17).

In some areas it might be possible to work out a 'take' rota, e.g. patients are allocated to nurses as they are admitted to a unit or team, with nurses taking it in turns both on a daily or shift-by-shift basis.

> We find, quite simply, that letting the staff determine the allocation of patients is a team decision. If a problem arises, then the charge nurse can always step in to make the decision if agreement cannot be reached, but in practice this never happened.
>
> *Senior primary nurse/charge nurse*

In the agreement, the principle should be that each patient should be able to identify his or her nurse for however long or short a time the patient's problem requires nursing care. Whether the patient arrives as a day case on the ward or is resident in a coronary care setting, or is requiring a limited number of visits in the community, then the goal is to achieve the 'my nurse' concept.

7.   How Do Nurses Make Themselves Known to Patients and Explain Primary Nursing?

Apart from the obvious but most important point of introducing oneself and explaining to the patient what primary nursing is all about, there are additional factors that can enhance patients' awareness of what is going on. After all, the patient may be disorientated or, with so many other things going on in his/her life at the time of illness in an unfamiliar setting, simply forgetful. In addition, other people need to know too: relatives, visitors, doctors, and other members of the multidisciplinary team. Wills and Wright (1988) identified the following possible features:

- The use of 'personal cards' (Figure 4.2), which can be given to patients or relatives.

> We have also produced identification cards for the primary nurses. We use a modification of the system used at Emory University Hospital, Atlanta (the link hospital in our international exchange system). The patient has one of these but they are useful for relatives too, to identify the nurse and provide an easy reference for the ward's telephone number.
>
> To start with, these are not particularly cheap to produce (about £170 per 3000 including artwork, etc.) but thereafter they cost about £30 per 1000. We consider this a worthwhile investment if it initiates understanding between nurse, patient and others and makes contact easier.
>
> *Primary nurse*

- At the entrance to the ward, a notice board can be set up that gives the names of the patients, their location on the ward, and the names of the primary/associate nurses caring for them. Photographs of the nursing staff, with names, can also be on display.
- Each ward can have an information centre for the use of both patients and relatives. Articles and information on primary nursing can be made available for staff, patients and relatives to read. Information leaflets (Figure 4.3, p. 66) for visitors to collect as they wish, can also be made available.

FRONT:

The Nursing Development Unit

Telephone:
Ask for Ward . . . .

. . . .   ו
Primary Nurse   Associate Nurse(s)

Caring for the Elderly

REVERSE:

You can expect your primary nurse to:
Get to know you and your family.
Plan with your doctor, for your care.
Plan with you the nursing care, to meet your needs.
Explain your needs to the associate nurse, who will care for you when your primary nurse is off duty.
Tell you what to expect before all tests or treatment.
Teach you about health care related to your condition.
Find the answers to your questions about your hospital stay.

We need you to:
Tell your primary nurse what you need.
Keep your nurse informed about how you feel and things that are on your mind.
Let your nurse know how you feel about the care you receive.
Tell your nurse if you have an idea or a preference about your nursing care.

Fig. 4.2   Example of a personal card

The Nursing Development Unit

Dear Visitor

Primary Nursing – what does it mean?

The Nursing Staff on the ward would like to tell you about our approach to nursing our patients – it's called 'Primary Nursing'.

Each patient has his or her own special nurse, called a 'Primary Nurse', who is the main person looking after the patient. An 'Associate Nurse' helps the Primary Nurse to give the care required.

When you visit our ward, look out for a photo of the 'Primary Nurse' with the 'Special Patient' and the information card telling you the name of the 'Special Nurse'. These are placed over the bed and on the notice board as you enter the ward.

For information about the patient you are visiting, or about Primary Nursing, please ask the Primary Nurse, who is the main care giver, or the Associate Nurse if he or she is not on duty. You might like to make a note of these nurses, so that you can ask for them if making a telephone enquiry.

We always welcome any comments regarding the nursing care of our patients: please let the Primary Nurse know your views. Alternatively you can write or telephone with your comments to the persons identified in the ward information book (at each patient's bedside) and on the 'comments and complaints' posters visible around the unit.

Thank you
The Nursing Staff

Caring for the Elderly

Fig. 4.3 Example of an information leaflet

The Nursing Development Unit

PATIENT'S NAME ....

THE TEAM OF STAFF CARING FOR YOU ARE:

PRIMARY NURSE   ....

ASSOCIATE NURSE   ....

....

CARE ASSISTANT   ....

DOCTOR   ....

OTHER THERAPISTS   ....

....

Fig 4.4 Bedside notice

- Photograph albums of the staff, giving information about their professional backgrounds, can be collated and made available for patients.
- Patients may be given a copy of the duty rota (where appropriate) relating to the team caring for them.
- A bedside notice illustrates 'who's who' (Figure 4.4).
- Another possibility is to have photographs of nurse and patient at the bedside:

> At the bedside on the continuing care wards, it is possible to have a photograph of both nurse and patient together, which can be attached to the head of the bed. This is not so easy on rapid turnover wards, but here we have found that simply a photograph of the nurse is sufficient. At the side of the picture is a name label giving the details of patient, primary nurse and associate nurse.
>
> *Primary nurse*

- Information books can also be given to patients.

> Each patient is given an information booklet. Apart from giving details on a variety of issues pertinent to his hospital stay, there is also a section describing primary nursing. The following is an extract from the booklet:
>
> *Nursing Care.* As often as possible the same nurses will be caring for you during your stay on the ward, so that you can get to know them and they can get to know you. You will be allocated your own special nurse, known as a 'primary nurse', who will be responsible for your nursing care throughout your stay. Your care will be discussed with you, and you are encouraged to read your nursing notes if you wish to. You will be asked if you would like your nursing notes to be kept at the bedside, or if you would prefer them to be kept at the nurses' station.
>
> *Associate nurse*

All of the above are merely adjuncts to effective nurse–patient communication; they are not a substitute for it. Making the roles of nurses in primary nursing clear to patients verbally on first contact, and repeating and reinforcing as necessary, are the most important. In this way, the primary nurse, for example, makes it very clear that 'I'm your nurse'.

Elements such as the 'personal cards' or 'photograph boards' are trappings which are designed to aid patient awareness of the system. They are not substitutes for it. Setting up a ward notice board of staff photographs does not mean that primary nursing has been implemented! In addition, different techniques will apply to different areas from wards to community. Above all, as Manthey (1970) suggests, the primary nurse is a 'visible' nurse who is known to the patient, the family and other disciplines.

8. What about Day-to-Day Organisation?

McFarlane and Castledine (1982) describe the pattern of care they used in one unit, which includes the following:

1. Each patient is allocated to a primary nurse for:
    *   assessing, planning, implementing and evaluating care;
    *   working with patients each time he/she is on duty;
    *   following patients' progress through hospitalisation;
    *   making home visits, e.g. before, during and after discharge;
    *   arranging transfer home;
    *   functioning as the patient's advocate;
    *   serving as the main co-ordinator of his total care;
    *   promoting his care at nursing care evaluation sessions.
2. Each patient is also allocated to a second (associate) nurse/student/nursing auxiliary, who helps to continue care both when the primary nurse is present and when he/she is away.
3. All nurses serve as associates to each other in the event of both primary and other associate nurse being absent.
4. Primary nurses attend case conferences, ward rounds, etc., when possible.
5. Primary nurse discusses changes to plan after days off, etc.

6. One nurse acts as overall ward co-ordinator on each shift (not necessarily ward sister/charge nurse).

The above illustrates one general approach to the organisation of primary nursing. Co-ordinating the staff in this way raises new difficulties. 'Off-duties' can be planned to ensure that 'care' is provided by both associate and primary nurse on rotation. These might actually look different from the usual 'off-duty' sheet (e.g. Figure 4.5).

In the example given in Figure 4.5, individual off-duties are organised to ensure sufficient 'cover' of staff and skill mixes during the course of the day. In other words, the off-duty is planned to ensure general trained staff cover of a particular unit, as well as ensuring that each group of patients retains their primary and associate nurses. Reorganising care along the lines of primary nursing can also bring about a change in the overall pattern of the patient's day. Traditionally, staffing levels tend to be planned with higher numbers in the morning and fewer in the evening. This may shift with primary nursing.

> We used to have six staff on in the morning and three or four in the evening (large, long-stay care of the elderly ward). Now, with the change of skill mix and the change in the pattern of the day, we need the numbers to be much more even – say 4/4 or 5/4.
>
> *Senior primary nurse/ward sister*

Changing the shift levels in one ward can, however, cause problems.

> Our ward ratios were different, but other wards working to the old pattern stayed the same. When someone went off sick (on the other wards), we began to feel like the loan-shop for the rest of the unit, i.e. we were seen to have higher than usual numbers of staff in the evening but, of course, they were there because they were needed. Other staff in other wards, though, can perceive you as being well off and therefore available for borrowing from.
>
> *Primary nurse*

OFF DUTY ROTA   WARD _____   WEEK COMMENCING _____

PLEASE PLACE CIRCLE AROUND NAME OF WARD CO-ORDINATOR (1st LEVEL NURSE) FOR EACH SHIFT

NAME	MONDAY	TUESDAY	WEDNESDAY	THURSDAY	FRIDAY	SATURDAY	SUNDAY
Primary Nurse							
Associate Nurse							
Associate Nurse							
Care Assistant							
Primary Nurse							
Associate Nurse							
Associate Nurse							
Care Assistant							
Primary Nurse							
Associate Nurse							
Associate Nurse							
Care Assistant							
Primary Nurse							
Associate Nurse							
Associate Nurse							
Care Assistant							
NIGHT DUTY							
Associate Nurse							
Associate Nurse							
Associate Nurse							
Care Assistant							
TOTAL WARD Nos.							

Fig. 4.5 'Off-duty' sheet

Another possibility to consider is flexible rostering. This can work on some units where the caseload is more erratic. For example, a day case surgical ward may organise their staff's hours to deal with planned admissions.

> I've been to one ward where they take lots of day cases. Some of the primary nurses took it in turns to adjust their hours, working from the time the patient came in, staying with them throughout their care during the day, until they went home. With flexible hours, they took the time back later.
>
> *Associate nurse*

In organising the day-to-day work of the ward, a variety of strategies can be tried as different options. In the end, what suits a particular setting best is that with which all staff and patients feel comfortable, and this can only be decided on an individual basis.

9.   What about Borrowing of Staff?

Primary nursing does not guarantee that nurses will not go off sick or that staffing crises do not occur (although it is argued that such incidents are reduced).

There can be problems when primary nursing is being implemented in some areas and not others.

> Our off-duties changed, that is the spread of staff over the day became different. We didn't have more staff, just deployed them differently. This meant we used to have three staff on duty in the evening where now we have four. The trouble is, other wards can see us as well staffed if their numbers fall. The pressure is on the borrower. They don't realise that the four staff are there because they are needed.
>
> *Primary nurse*

Primary nursing need not mean that staff become inflexible or unresponsive to the wider sense of the team which exists on the larger unit. Helping each other out is an essential consequence when problems arise. However, it does place an issue firmly before management: look at a whole range of strategies to reduce the problem and not just manage the crisis by shunting staff around.

> I had a terrible incident one evening. It left me quaking in my shoes! The nurse manager wanted to borrow one of my staff. I didn't refuse at first and tried to get him to look at how we could help without major depletion of our staff (i.e. we could have adjusted our working pattern in the short term to help 'cover' for meals, etc.). In the end, I had to point out the care planning and the allocation of patients, and the workload. I told him, 'If you take this primary nurse, then six patients will have no-one to care for them. Would you please sign in the notes that you will accept responsibility if anything goes wrong or if there is a complaint!'. I told him that 'We will cope if we have to, I can't *stop* you enforcing your decision, but if you do, I want it in writing'. I thought, this is it – the sack! He went white and just left the ward. Then I felt really awful, not just for myself, but for the other ward which I knew must be really stuck, but I told myself: 'My priority is my patients, my code of conduct tells me that there's no point in robbing Peter to pay Paul'. How did it end? He called someone in on overtime!
>
> *Senior primary nurse/ward sister*

Borrowing and moving of staff has become an accepted activity in nursing because nurses will 'cope'. It should be seen as a last resort when all other strategies have failed. It is not a problem unique to primary nursing, and it is short changing patients wherever and whenever it occurs. What primary nursing seems to do is to thrust the difficulty into sharp focus. When considered with the skills of the questioning assertive nurse, then the manager's role is also tested. Is support for primary nursing merely lip-service or is there really a creative management approach evident? Issues like staffing problems are one of the ways in which this is tested.

It also has to be said that the borrowing of staff does not mean that primary nursing has collapsed. In the short term, it may be no more than an irritant or frustration that niggles at the clinical nurse who has to work around it.

However, if it becomes consistent and long term, it may undermine the whole practice of primary nursing, which depends at least upon a reasonably reliable deployment of staff. Primary nurses and their colleagues cannot continue in their role when they are dogged by constant uncertainties of who their patients will be. The expectations of the patients are also not fulfilled in such circumstances. The occasional 'slip' in staffing levels – a ward or small unit when staff and patients are well known to each other – can easily be managed. If it becomes a permanent problem, it must be questioned whether efforts to maintain primary nursing can be continued, because of the risks of exhaustion and frustration to the staff and the conflicting messages being given to patients. In the long term, primary nursing requires reasonable stability in the nursing workforce. When this is not happening, then questions must be asked, beyond primary nursing, about what is going wrong and keeps nurses out of commitment to nursing, and what can be done to put things right.

10.   What Reporting Methods Are Necessary?

If the basis of primary nursing is that of a working partnership with the patient, then this will require a shift away from traditional reporting methods (i.e. the staff gathered separately from patients at 'hand-over' time). In the Nursing Developing Unit at Tameside the following methods have proved effective:

- Each primary or associate nurse gives a verbal and written report on his/her group of patients.
- All staff are involved in a general 'walk round' of the ward at report handover times (e.g. between two shifts) to receive the verbal report. This ensures that all staff have a working knowledge of all patients. They can still therefore render effective help to all patients, e.g. in the sudden absence of the primary/associate nurse or simply 'in passing'. Primary nursing does not mean that the allocated nurses attend only to 'my patients' and

ignore all others! The staff still have to work as a team. Clearly, such reporting methods need to be used sensitively, to ensure patient confidentiality. One of the main purposes of the bedside handover is the oppor- tunity for nurse and patient to meet each other. It may be inappropriate in some settings for intimate details of patient care to be exchanged at this stage.

- Patients' nursing records are kept at the bedside (if they choose) and reports are made with the patient at the bedside. The patient may write in the notes if he or she wishes. Of course, the patient will not be disturbed for note writing while asleep.
- The patient is involved in discussion on his or her care at report times by the team. These tend to be very general discussions so that confidentiality is not breached within earshot of the patients. Detailed aspects of care can be discussed separately between individual nurses transferring care of the patient, and between nurse and patient.
- Access to nursing notes by patients is decided using the strategy shown in the 'case study' below.
- Nursing notes are filed with medical records after discharge. Photocopies of the care plans, etc., can be given to the patient to hand to his or her community nurse where appropriate.

Case study

Comments on confidentiality with reference to access to notes by patients

1. The notes relate to *nursing* notes and not medical notes – specifically the content of care plans, assessment sheets and evaluation.
2. The basic assumption is that the patient has the right of access to the information with the right to comment on the content.
3. The primary nurse bears the responsibility for explaining *all* the implications to the patient of having access to notes, particularly in relation to matters of confidentiality, specifically:
   - An absolute guarantee of confidentiality cannot be made if

continued next page

continued _____

> notes are kept at the bedside (i.e. may be accessible for other patients, visitors or family to read without the patient's consent.)
> - Potential problems can be minimised by following the suggested guidelines on access (See Figure 4.6, p. 78).
> - Notes can be retained by the patient, either in the patient's locker or at the head of the bed, giving closer possession within the patient's personal space.
>
> 4. All nurses must be fully aware of and skilled in completing nursing notes unambiguously and objectively as they may be asked to justify written phrases by the patient (and his family).
> 5. All nurses should read and fully understand the guidelines discussed in the UKCC advisory paper, specifically:
>   - The paragraph (clause nine) that reads:
>   'Each registered nurse, midwife and health visitor is accountable for his or her practice, and in the exercise of professional accountability shall respect confidential information obtained in the course of professional practice and refrain from disclosing such information *without the consent* of the patient/client, or a person entitled to act on his/her behalf, except where disclosure is required by law or by order of a court or is necessary in the public interest.'
>   - In general, information on patients might be disclosed under a number of categories, among which is:
>
>   *'With the consent of the patient/client'*
>
>   Clearly this category does not constitute a breach of confidentiality, since consent implies that the patient's autonomy has been respected.
> 6. The patient's informed consent, once given, must be clearly documented/dated and signed by the nurse responsible.
>
> **General points relating to patients' access to nursing notes**
>
> 1. Patients' access to notes must be monitored continuously by the nurse in charge of the patient as part of the total programme of care.
> 2. Notes and care plans must be checked and reviewed daily by the primary nurse (or associate in his/her absence).
> 3. Contents of notes, when left at the bedside, must be reviewed with and explained to the patient by the nurse responsible for his/her care.
> 4. When in doubt, keep the nursing notes at the nurses' station until reviewed and discussed by the primary nurse with appropriate colleagues.
>
> *continued next page*

continued

> 5. The primary nurse should discuss 'sensitive' issues, i.e. dying or sexualising and the patient's degree of acceptance, with more senior colleagues when necessary, before leaving the notes with the patient.
> 6. The patient's choice of access should be recorded in the nursing notes, particularly if consent has been given.
> 7. All patients' care plans are discussed with the patient by the nurse in charge of their care, regardless of their choice to retain the notes or not.
> 8. Patients' personal choices must be adhered to and respected at all times.
> 9. Any care plan or evaluation completed by a student nurse must be checked and countersigned by the registered nurse.
> 10. All potential primary nurses and practising primary nurses should improve and widen their knowledge basis in this area and must attend the appropriate training packages on the unit.
> 11. Patients are to be actively encouraged to read, comment upon, question the content of and write in their care plan if they wish to do so.

Patient access to health care information has been embodied in British law since 1990. The Patient's Charter (DoH, 1991) reinforces this right. Individual patients will vary greatly in the way they will wish to have access to their records and the degree of involvement in care. For some it will be of immediate significance, while others will consider it irrelevant (but may change their minds later). It is essential that nurses are flexible and adaptable enough to adopt different approaches with different patients at different times. Waterman and Luker (1990) and Biley (1989, 1991) reinforce the view that involving patients in care, including access to health records, is highly problematic. It is important that nurses deal with the issue sensitively. In working from the basic principle that patients have the right of access and involvement if they choose to do so, it is then possible to adopt a variety of approaches which include individual patients' needs. Just as the patients have 'my nurse', they may also wish to have 'my records'. However, without adequate support and advice, involving patients in care could become just

PATIENT ADMITTED – OFFERED CHOICE OF KEEPING NOTES AT BEDSIDE/NURSES' STATION – IMPLICATIONS EXPLAINED

If chooses to keep at bedside	Wants to see notes but not keep them at bedside	Does not wish to keep notes	Unable to make choice (e.g. disorientated/ unconscious)
a. Explain full implications and confidentiality issues	(e.g. does not wish relatives to see them)	Explain that notes will be stored at the nurses' station	a. Explain that notes will be retained at the nurses' station where appropriate
b. Record/date/sign when consent has been given in the nursing notes	Offer to let patient see notes on a daily basis or as requested by patient, e.g. at report-writing time	a. Discuss contents of the plans with patient at the bedside	b. Follow personal request of patient's close relatives (who have given all the details for assessment)
Keeping nursing notes in a secure place with the patient, i.e. locker/bedhead	a. Discuss contents of plans with patient at bedside	b. Retain notes at the nurses' station	c. Primary nurse may choose to make decision for patient (if no relatives) and remain fully accountable/ responsible for decision
Discuss contents of plans with patient at bedside	b. Retain notes at the nurses' station	Patient may write in evaluation if he or she wishes	d. Record/date/sign final decision in patient's notes
a. Patient may write in evaluations if wishes	Patient may write in evaluation if he or she wishes	Check at regular intervals to see if patient wishes to change mind (e.g. originally felt 'too ill' to bother and now improving)	When condition improves, discuss contents with patient and relatives at bedside
b. Check at regular intervals if patient is still happy about retaining notes	Check at regular intervals for change of mind, if patient wishes to keep notes		Review with patient when able to make rational choice

Access to notes

Fig. 4.6 Guidelines on access to nursing notes by patients another ritual and routine. Nurses need to be able to respond accordingly to different needs and approaches from different patients.

11. How Do Student and Pupil Nurses Fit into the Scheme?

(Please refer to question 8 above and to Chapter 2.)

The student nurse is not a qualified nurse and cannot act as a primary nurse. He or she may work as associate nurse, but should have duty rotas organised so that constant supervision is maintained. The degree of involvement in care will vary according to the student's level of experience and ability. It is part of the role of the primary nurse to be a teacher/supporter of others. Indeed, primary nursing seems to facilitate this in line with the ENB (1987a) recommendations on the provision of 'mentoring' for students. McDermott (1992) suggests that the student's experience in primary nursing can be a very positive one.

The evaluations by students of their stay here (primary nursing ward) are rated really high. They have a much richer experience working with this ratio and a manageable group of patients. They seem to learn to manage the nurse–patient relationship better, get a more in-depth knowledge of the patient and his or her problems and are better able to develop and transfer their theoretical knowledge into practice.

Clinical teacher

When the primary nurse or mentor is not on duty, the other primary nurses can ensure that students are helped and adequately supervised.

For the first time, I felt I was learning to nurse here. I found it was better to get to know a few in depth rather than a lot superficially. I felt like part of the team and got to understand better about involvement with patients and how we can work 'with' them rather than 'at' them.

Student nurse

Organising the workload with students remains a permanent problem when they are still allocated as part of the workforce. Students allocated under P2000 schemes for clinical experience are usually not included as part of the workforce, and their opportunities for support within primary nursing teams are considerably enhanced.

12.   Can Primary Nursing Work on Night Duty?

Yes. The roles need to be carefully worked through and joint meetings of staff arranged to identify working patterns. In general, it is very difficult for the night nurse to be a primary nurse because of the more restricted access to the multidisciplinary team, relatives or other carers. Again, it is important that the roles are clearly understood and valued. Being the associate nurse does not mean that the role is any less valuable than the primary nurse, nor does it mean that independent decisions about care cannot be made, or initial assessments and plans of care completed. It is also necessary to distinguish between primary nursing continuing on night duty (i.e. the organisational method/philosophy of care is maintained) and there not being a primary nurse on night duty.

Much depends on the factors in each setting, e.g. whether internal rotation of day/night staff is feasible either for all or some of the staff, the number of part-time staff, skill mixes and so on. It is therefore difficult to lay down hard and fast rules; each setting is unique and must decide for itself the way forward. Certainly, where there is continuity of staff on nights in a unit and if, for example, the greater part of the patient's nursing problems are at night, there is no reason why the night nurse cannot act as the primary nurse.

Where a system of internal rotation of staff, between days and nights, is in operation, a decision will have to be made whether or not the primary nurse remains in that role on night duty. The following will need to be considered:

- the length of time the night duty period lasts;
- whether or not the primary nurse can still maintain

co-ordination and continuity of care satisfactorily from a night duty position. This will vary depending on the nurse's hours of work, patient needs, and so on;

- whether the associate nurse coming on to day duty changes to a primary nursing role;
- how the changes are explained to patients and others who are affected.

The following case study illustrates some of these issues:

Case study

INTRODUCING PRIMARY NURSING TO NIGHT DUTY

As the night sister allocated to the ward, I was eager to learn as much as possible about primary nursing. This I did by reading papers and articles on the subject, including the ones produced by the staff on Ward X where primary nursing had already been introduced, discussions with other nursing staff and attending a conference on primary nursing.

For the day staff primary nursing was also a new innovation, so I felt this was the ideal opportunity for the day and night staff to improve their relationship with one another and break down the day/night barrier while improving the continuity of care given to the patient. I approached the introduction of primary nursing to night duty in the following way:

- Many of the night staff I discussed primary nursing with were very pessimistic that it could be implemented successfully, while others were totally opposed to the idea. A minority were enthusiastic and eager to gain further information on the topic; these were the staff I was hoping would be allocated to the ward!
- Because of the mixed reaction I received from the staff I decided it was the appropriate time to approach the night nurse manager to discuss the necessity of a stable night team, who were interested and motivated, to be allocated to the ward. The nurse manager was already aware of the impending arrival of primary nursing as I had ensured that she was informed of all up to date developments. She gave me her full support as far as possible but could not guarantee that the same team of nurses would always be allocated to the ward. This I was aware would be one of the greatest problems.
- I liaised closely with the day staff and attended meetings to discuss implementation of primary nursing and the role the night staff would play. The need for improved communication between day and night staff was paramount if we were to be successful.

continued next page

continued

- Many of the night staff found it difficult to attend meetings held by the day staff. I acted as their representative. The information I received was then related to other members of the night nursing team and we discussed ideas on the best way to approach primary nursing from a night point of view. In turn, key members of staff on days agreed to short spells of night duty, and meetings were held at night which day staff attended.
- I made a point of educating my colleagues about primary nursing. Literature was made available on the ward. I ensured I was available if the staff wished to discuss the subject. I also encouraged the staff to attend any courses or conferences relating to primary nursing.
- It was agreed with the day staff that the night nurse would on the whole take the role of associate nurse. In the event of the majority of problems a particular patient encountered occurring at night, then the RGN on night duty would take the role of primary nurse for the patient.
- The staff allocated to the ward at night often consists of an RGN, an SEN and a nursing auxiliary. Usually the RGN gives all of the report in hand-over time to the day staff. This changed as each trained nurse reported on his/her own patients.
- I also felt it important that the idea of the night staff carrying out a short spell on day duty, and vice versa, would be encouraged so that all problems would be appreciated by all members of the nursing staff. Communication between staff would be improved, leading to an improved 24-hour service for the patient.
- A white board was provided for ward use to enable the staff to specify which patients they were caring for. The night staff have been added to this board and each was allocated a group of patients for whom they acted as associate nurse. The nurse acted as associate nurse for at least one spell of duty, i.e. three/four nights, if necessary, if the patient's length of stay was greater. (This was an acute ward – average length of stay for most patients was 7 days.)
- I found that the approach to primary nursing at night must be flexible and it will alter depending upon the ward situation and staffing levels. Each trained staff nurse acted as associate nurse for 12 patients, with the auxiliary nurse taking the role of aide or helper. The associate nurse carries out the care prescribed, writes the nursing notes and gives a report on her patients to the day staff, discussing any appropriate change of care with the primary nurse.

Night sister

Kemp's (1992) research identifies many of the difficulties which night nurses face – including the effects of isolation from the mainstream of the organisation, physiological and psychological effects, reduced opportunities for education, and so on. Involving night staff in the whole team approach to primary nursing is essential. Some of the following points may be helpful:

- Night nurses should be involved in all stages of development and planning of primary nursing. Establishing regular ward meetings at flexible times (alternately at times convenient to day and night staff) will create an ideal forum for issues to be discussed.
- An overlap of shifts can be arranged or an exchange of shifts between day and night staff can be organised. This can help to demolish barriers and friction between team members. The recent development of the G grade's role suggests that the senior co-ordinator can be on night duty regularly. This ensures recognition of the need for information and support to be passed on over a 24-hour basis.
- Written information is available for all night nurses by offering access to nursing journals and books on primary nursing. Open learning packs should also be available for staff to work through at their own pace, and perhaps a library and resource centre established offering a variety of books, projects, videotapes, and so on, which is accessible to all staff 24 hours a day.
- Teaching on night duty:
  - A clinical nurse specialist nurse, nurse teacher or other facilitator can organise specific teaching sessions or courses relevant to the needs of night nurses.
  - Initiating 'lunch-time' teaching for nurses during the night.
  - Use of open learning packs, videotapes.
  - Organising more evening/weekend workshops where night nurses can also attend.
  - Provide time out/study leave to attend study days/ visit units/do degree courses.

Nursing on night duty can be difficult under any circumstances and the changes brought about by primary nursing can produce many threats and uncertainties. With the application of some of the principles suggested above, the path can be made much smoother.

There are therefore many implications for night staff in primary nursing. Remington (1989) notes: 'It would be a great mistake to see primary nursing as just the latest in a line of nursing fads that came in with a bang and go out with a whimper. Permanent night staff must be aware of what the concept entails and what the implications will be for them'.

The strength of the team, as suggested earlier, appears to be crucial in determining night staff involvement in, and commitment to, primary nursing. The issues are often emotive and revolve around feelings of status and being valued. Joint meetings, internal rotation, occasional exchange of shifts from days to nights and vice versa can all help to consolidate a team spirit, remove the sense of isolation that so often bedevils night nursing and help build up a collegial relationship of mutual trust and understanding.

13.   Can the Care Assistant or Support Worker Be a Primary or Associate Nurse?

Primary nursing is clearly a role designated for the qualified nurse, and, as has been suggested earlier, the associate may be a student nurse under certain circumstances. The care assistant/nursing auxiliary role is designed to assist the nurse to deliver care effectively (see Chapter 3). However, conflicts can arise if the care assistants are not fully included as members of the team, and McFarlane and Castledine (1982) seem to suggest that they can be included as associates. They too have a vital role to play in promoting the 'primary nursing culture' and the sense of team spirit. They can, for example, still be involved in decisions which affect the unit and its policies, and particularly their own working practices. Working in teams with primary and associate nurses, they can retain supervised patient contact and continue to contribute through their help with, and observations on, patients and their care.

> As a nursing auxiliary on this unit I am as much a part of the team as everyone else. I take part in all the reporting sessions, and help the primary nurse with her patients. If I notice something about a patient, then I would tell her. I write things I notice in the nursing notes too.
>
> *Care assistant/nursing auxiliary, Elderly Care Unit*

It is essential that the degree of involvement and purpose in nursing is recognised, otherwise the nursing auxiliary/ care assistant can feel relegated to the role of mere kitchen cleaner and not an overall helper in care. In many settings nursing auxiliaries have been major care-givers, and some may not relish the return of their true role. Sadly, this has occurred not because of a flaw in primary nursing, but because of failings in nursing as a whole. The nursing auxiliary should never have been led into a position where he or she is the assessor, planner, giver and evaluator of care, which has occurred in some settings. This is an abuse of the nursing auxiliary and an infringement of the patient's right to skilled nursing. As primary nursing develops, especially when the skill mix is changed, then the role of the true helper to the nurse and patient must emerge. The care assistant/nursing auxiliary should not be placed in a position where he or she replaces the trained nurse. Inevitably, some nursing auxiliaries can feel a sense of loss if required to adopt their true role, while others will feel more comfortable at having their role more clearly defined – and not doing more than that which they are paid to do!

> Things were changing generally on the unit, not just primary nursing. Inevitably, some of the auxiliaries left because they didn't like not being 'in
>
> *continued next page*

continued

charge' any more, but most fitted well into the new scheme of things. I felt
sorry for those who felt unable to adapt. After all, it was our fault
historically that had led them into a role for which they were not properly
prepared or being rewarded. We encouraged quite a number to get into
nurse training themselves – if they were that good they should be trained
and paid for it.

Nurse manager

Many nursing auxiliaries and others have now trained as
'support workers' under the NVQ system (Chapter 3),
which enables them to carry out many tasks previously
considered to be the remit of nurses. That all staff should
have access to better training to national standards would
appear to have many all-round benefits. How far can those
with higher levels of training be included within the
primary nursing system? Without appropriate professional
accountability, the necessary knowledge base for decision-
making, independent assessing, planning, giving and
evaluating of care and so on, it would not be appropriate
for the 'support workers' to work as primary nurses. In
addition, the title 'nurse' can only apply in law to someone
who has completed a recognised qualification and whose
name appears on the register of nurses.

Certain aspects of care, according to the level of training, can be delegated providing supervision is available.
The primary nurse, as the qualified nurse, remains
responsible for ensuring that anyone participating in the
care of his/her patients is competent to deliver the care
required. The primary nurse also remains accountable for
any such delegated aspects of care, and the support worker
is responsible to the primary nurse for any care he/she
gives. In some settings, support workers have been used to
replace associate nurses as associate carers. They may care
for a group of patients in the absence of the primary nurse,
but remain supervised by another qualified colleague. It is
questionable whether such an approach is appropriate to
primary nursing, bearing in mind the issues discussed

about accountability and the value of nursing practice as discussed in Chapter 3.

14. Doesn't Primary Nursing Reinforce the Élitist Position of the Primary Nurse?

Previous sections of this chapter have emphasised the need for a strong team and collegial spirit to promote primary nursing. Élites already exist in ward and community hierarchies. Primary nursing is not about élitism; it is about matching nurses to patients so that the patient gets the quality of care to which he or she has right. Even the word 'primary' has a superior ring to it, being equated with the Latin word 'primus', meaning first. However, arguing over terminology would be a sterile debate. What matters more is the attitude of all nurses in the team, which recognises and values the roles of each other in meeting the patients' needs for care. The primary nurse is not necessarily the best person, but because of his or her knowledge and skill should be the best placed to solve the patient's nursing problems by functioning as a primary nurse. Thus the primary nurse is not an élitist, but a thinking-doer, putting skills to the use of the patient and working with colleagues towards that central function.

15. What about the Medical and Other Staff?

Traditionally, in the hospital setting, when other disciplines have wanted information about a patient, they have tended to approach the ward sister or charge nurse. With autonomy and accountability devolved to each primary nurse, there is a risk of confusion, if not hostility!

Responses in the studies seem to have been very varied. McFarlane and Castledine (1982) reported that 'our doctors just find it a little strange that, instead of consulting the ward sister about each patient, they had to relate more to the rest of the trained staff'. The 'visibility' notice suggested earlier appears to be as helpful to doctors as to nurses and patients. A programme of education of medical staff may be as important as that for the nurses. Responses may vary from (a) pleasure of many medical and other disciplines with the increased collaboration which occurs, to (b) others who have found primary nursing threatening because they are 'not in charge of nurses' (Hegyvary, 1982). As Hugman (1991) illustrates, 'the language of professionalism frequently serves to obscure the issue of power'. The experience of the Nursing Development Unit illustrates the following principal issues:

- Most members of other disciplines were, in practice, very supportive. They saw primary nursing as mirroring their own practice in some ways, and as having trained staff responsible for individual patients.
- The multidisciplinary team, as well as patients and relatives, have to be involved in the run-up to primary nursing. Explaining what it is all about and giving plenty of time for questions, involvement in unit meetings, trial periods, reassessments, and so on, will encourage co-operation.
- 'Selling' primary nursing to other disciplines was important in that they not only understood it, but could see advantages in it for them, i.e. they would know that a particular nurse had an in-depth knowledge of a particular patient, would be better able to assist them, and could be specifically identified (e.g. as opposed to 'passing the buck') when a problem of continuity of care arose.
- Being prepared for role conflicts, most specifically with some medical staff who have become accustomed to (and might prefer!) the ward sister or hand-maiden and fount of all knowledge about patients.
- Demonstrating that the quality of care has improved (e.g. from the results of quality assurance tests used).
- Demonstrating that other staff can have confidence in other nurses previously considered 'junior'.
- Showing how the application of primary nursing is essential to meeting wider organisational/managerial objectives, i.e. the application of the national 'named

nurse' (DoH, 1991) policy. (See also the discussion on 'the doctor–nurse game' in Chapter 6.)

> Some of the doctors were hesitant at first, but it depends on how you manage the situation. We spent time explaining what it was all about beforehand. But in the end, there's nothing like experience for learning. Other professionals began to learn that they could trust the primary nurse simply because they experienced her knowledge and skills in relation to the patient. In some settings, colleagues adapted very quickly; in others it took longer to overcome the doubts. The ward sister/charge nurse's approach is particularly important in helping to wean the other disciplines away from complete dependence on him or her and in encouraging them to accept the new organisation. After a while, we were surprised how few problems we had in this area. We even had doctors coming back and telling us how surprised they were with the nurse's knowledge of the patient! The relationships began to change quite significantly.
>
> *Senior primary nursing/ward sister*

Some problems can also occur for the sisters/charge nurses themselves (see earlier in the chapter) as they have to cope with the perception of other disciplines about the role. These perceptions of roles are discussed at length by Argyle (1978), who notes that conflict and 'role strain' may come from three main sources. It may arise between roles (for example, the working nurse who is also a wife and mother) or within a role (for example, the ward sister who must be both primary nurse and ward manager, yet the two may not always overlap easily). A third source is the conflict which occurs in the 'role set', the people nurses work with day to day who have different roles from the nurse and who have different perspectives on what nursing is. The ward sister/charge nurse's role set, for example, would include patients, doctors, ward nursing colleagues, relatives and nurse manager.

To minimise such stresses and strains around the role of primary nurse, it is, therefore, essential that non-nursing colleagues are also prepared for what primary nursing is. That is not to say that nurses need, for example, to ask the doctors *if* they can start primary nursing. Rather, as colleagues in the multidisciplinary team, they should have the concept explained to them so that when the change begins they are less likely to meet resistance and hostility.

16.   What Happens if the Patient is Transferred to a Non-primary Nursing Area?

Primary nurses can accompany the patient to that ward or the patient's home, or a nurse who will be allocated to that patient may pay a visit to meet the patient first. Primary nursing tends to raise expectations for patients, which may not be met in other areas where primary nursing is not being practised. Clearly, there has to be a very careful preparation of the patient beforehand if there is awareness that organisation of care may be different in another area; then the patient will find this less threatening.

> In some ways we've found this a positive thing. The expectation of patients has led the ward to look at their organisation of the care and use us for advice. Of course, there have been others who are just not ready for it and have shunned the very idea. It's important that the patient is aware that things may be a little different, and also not to imply that his care will be any the worse.
>
> *Primary nurse*

In the case of patients who are readmitted to a primary nursing area, it may well be that they return to the care of the previous primary nurse. Again, there should be no hard and fast rule about this. A degree of flexibility is needed to take account of factors such as the patient's and nurse's wishes, the length of the referral before readmission, the nature of the patient's renewed problems, and so on. The team need to make an early decision in the light of these factors, what is in the patient's best interests and, of course, what the patient's wishes are. In general, to promote continuity of care, it is desirable that the same patients have the same nurses where possible.

17. Perhaps the Patient and I Will Not 'Get On', or Maybe all this Closeness Will Be Too Much of a Strain – How Does the Nurse Manage this Close Contact with Patients?

There is nothing in primary nursing that suggests that every nurse must like every patient and vice versa. However, it is the experience of the team contributing to this book that difficulties associated with working with some patients are greatly diminished. This could be due to a variety of factors, for example:

- The presence of a supportive team of colleagues as a precursor to and continual requirement of primary nursing.
- The shift in emphasis of working with the patient and family as patients/companions.

'Difficult' patients are often labelled 'unpopular' (Stockwell, 1972) because they are demanding of the nurse's time and energy. Much of the basis for this lies in the patient's fears and insecurities, which, if the nurse is working freely with the patient as helper and information giver, can be greatly reduced.

Reports by the Health Service Ombudsman (1986–1993) seem to indicate that the majority of patients' complaints centre around inadequate communication skills. In primary nursing, keeping the patients informed, explaining, teaching and taking account of their views are an integral part of their care. How many nurses have been told not to 'get involved' with patients? As has been suggested earlier, primary nursing is all about being 'involved', so that the patients (and relatives and other carers too) are in a position to be active participants in care.

> At first we thought of dividing the patients up into 'our' groups. We agreed that, if any nurse was having conflict with a patient, then we could swap. In practice it just never happened. Some patients seemed less 'difficult', perhaps because they had developed more secure relationships with us.
>
> *Primary nurse*

> When I was working in the long stay areas, I thought this would really be a problem. So much so that, when we were 'starting out' we agreed to change our assignments after 3 months if necessary. We simply couldn't envisage wanting to stay with the same group of patients (or them with us). Of course, it just never happened! Something changes in the way you work with patients. The continuity of the relationship, and the rewards which come from that, seem to become more important than the change of scene.
>
> *Primary nurse*

The assumption is often made that the nurse will need a change of patients. Primary nursing calls this into question. Of course, there is also the corollary that the patient may wish to make a change too! In general, both circumstances should be extremely rare. The writers have all been primary nurses where many thousands of patients have passed through our care. Although the proviso was made that nurse and patient could change assignments, this happened only once in 10 years. (In this instance, a patient refused to have any contact with a particular nurse. The ward then discussed the problem, and the nurse herself felt she should be reassigned because of the risk of the added stress to the patient.) Allowing nurses and patients always to choose who shall have whom is extremely problematic, and is fraught with ethical dilemmas. Supposing the patient refuses a nurse on the grounds of colour prejudice? Supposing a nurse refuses a patient because of his/her illness (e.g. an AIDS patient)? In British law, nurses have no rights to refuse care and patients, while having many rights to choose in health care may find there are limits to such choices (Gooch, 1992; RCN, 1993b). Clearly, any therapeutic relationship is undermined if there is hostility between nurse and patient, and every case will have to be handled individually and sensitively. There is no hard and fast rule that a nurse and patient must be allocated to one another and remain together. However, where problems occur, the reasons need to be very carefully explored. Breaking the relationship between nurse and patient should be seen as a last resort.

The approach to assignment needs to remain open and flexible, as follows:

- There need to be no hard and fast rules about length of assignment. Experience has shown that, despite fears to the contrary, the nurses themselves will not, ultimately, put a time limit on it.

- Added stress for the nurse can be produced when the patient is more demanding, i.e. in need of more physical or psychological attention; and the patient's dependency level is greater. Thus, primary nurses' caseloads should not be fixed. Some nurses might have seven patients, others three, in the same unit. The level needs to be determined by the needs of patients. Conflicts with patients may often arise because the nurse is not fulfilling the role with all patients because of an overstretched caseload.

- While the primary nurse is accountable for the patient's care over 24 hours, it does not mean that he/she is 'on call' 24 hours a day! The associate nurse is an accountable trained nurse too and should not normally need to seek help from the primary nurse outside normal working hours. When help is needed, there will normally be other primary/senior nurses available to assist. However, if the primary nurse wishes to be involved, then there is no reason why this should not be so.

> Being called up at home is an extremely rare occurrence. It happened a few times on this ward in the past few years. It might be because the primary nurse has overlooked something important and the associate nurse needs to call her to check. However, it's more likely that the primary nurse herself has asked to be called. I can think of one instance when a patient, with no known relatives, was dying. The primary nurse asked to be called if anything happened during the night.
>
> *Senior primary nurse/ward sister*

- Managing the nurse–patient relationship in nursing requires a supportive team of colleagues in any circumstances. This is no less so in primary nursing. Flexibility with rules in relation to workload and length of assignment is essential. In practice, changing nurses and patients will be a rare event. A climate that allows nurses to express their feelings about patients is also needed – which does not criticise nurses who become upset because a patient dies, or censure them because they are having difficulty managing a patient's problems. If close contact is more demanding of nurses, this cannot be countenanced without the right climate to support the nurses.

- In relation to the above point, if nurses become more involved with patients, then clearly both nurse and patient may need to have new strategies to help them cope with separation when the time comes. For example, it may be possible for the patient to have the opportunity to telephone or visit the ward after discharge to follow up any queries, seek advice or just say 'thank you'. For the nurse, it may be important to have a chance to say 'goodbye' to a patient, especially if he or she is moving elsewhere or the patient is being discharged from care. It is important that the team encourages nurses to express their feelings and supports them when they do. Do the effects of separation support criticism of primary nursing? It may be argued that where roles and accountability are clearer, and team support in place, then nurses may find termination of the nurse–patient relationship less stressful than otherwise.

- *Patient contact hours.* Most authors agree that the relationship between nurse and patient is easier to develop where the patient is in for a longer stay. What about the short term? Manthey (1980) has this to say:

'Since the patient will be receiving some nursing during his short stay, I see no reason why he should not know the name of the nurse responsible for that care. Someone will be making some kind of decisions'.

She goes on to argue that:

> 'It may not be necessary to have a nursing care plan for the short-term patient, but primary nursing is visible responsibility for decision making, not the existence of elaborate care plans'.

In addition, staff who work part time or as 'bank nurses' are affected by their limitations of contact hours with the patient. Whether or not the part-time nurse is a primary nurse will depend upon the number of hours worked and the length of stay of the patient.

• Primary nursing is also not necessarily synonymous with documentation/care planning. It could be argued, however, that care planning tends to improve where nurses have their own group of patients and hence only their own care plans to deal with. Many nurses might ask how they can be expected to primary nurse when they seem to have little time as it is to plan care! Of course, the two are related, yet remain separate. Manthey (1988a) notes succinctly:

> 'Primary nursing is not synonymous with care plans! Primary nursing requires that each patient know the name of his or her primary nurse. Primary nursing also requires that each primary nurse be responsible for giving and co-ordinating whatever care the patient receives during the hospital stay. With short-term patients, primary nurses learn to perform short-term, realistic assessments and set short-term, realistic goals. Whether care plans are written is a separate issue of communication and/or documentation'.

Thus, whether it be in operating theatres or casualty departments, the principles of primary nursing can still apply. A named nurse, known to the patient, can be allocated, no matter how short the time. In fact it might be argued that in high-activity areas (often associated with a great deal of threat to the patients), having a reassuring person to whom the patient can relate is even more essential (see question 23).

18.   Do Tasks Disappear?

Not necessarily. What might be called 'housekeeping' duties are clearly the role of the care assistant, to enable the trained nurse to get on with the job of nursing. At other times, better use might be made of the ward clerk or secretarial role. Functions such as managing the ward budget, re-ordering stores, planning off-duties, etc., can either be delegated to ward clerks (in some settings these have become ward 'managers' or 'co-ordinators') or dispersed in rotation among the staff.

> In general, everybody seems to hate doing the non-nursing jobs like checking the linen supplies or planning the off-duty. We made sure that some jobs were clearly the work of the assistants; we focused on the nursing. The assistants would then also help us with things that needed two persons (e.g. lifting) as well as helping each other.
>
> We also delegated things like off-duty planning, ordering stores, etc., among ourselves, e.g. one nurse would do the off-duties for a month, another the store checking, and so on. It also meant that each member of staff had some experience in these things.
>
> *Senior primary nurse/charge nurse*

Sometimes it seems more difficult to escape the tasks because they are bound up in hospital procedure and policy books, although these are less common.

> Medicines used to be carried out by a strict two-person procedure. Eventually, we obtained a new medicine trolley with individual dispensers. Each patient's medicines were contained in a separate box, topped up by the pharmacist each day. The primary nurse could simply take medicines from the box labelled for each patient without having to take the whole trolley. That way each primary or associate nurse saw to it that 'their' patients got their medicines. We managed to get rid of the 'round'.
>
> *Primary nurse*

Activities that are focused on the patient are carried out by the primary/associate nurse for that patient. Dividing patients up into neatly packaged procedures (the 'temps', the 'BPs', the 'dressings') is incompatible with primary nursing.

19. What about Primary Nursing in the Community?

The principles of primary nursing are universal. Manthey (1988a) describes the concept of 'my nurse: my neighbour'. The question is an organisational one. Primary (community) nurses have a caseload of patients and address themselves to the patients' nursing needs as a whole.

> Each nurse in the clinic took his or her own caseload of patients. Sometimes we worked flexi hours if, say, the patient required some aspect of care in the evening. Otherwise, an associate nurse would go in, but the overall planning and co-ordination of care remain with the primary nurse.
>
> *Primary nurse in community care*

In many respects, community nursing has tended to retain many elements of Nightingale's 'case method' approach. However, community based care runs a risk of being fragmented equal to that of hospital based care. It is true that much of the writing on primary nursing has tended to focus on the hospital setting. Perhaps this is not surprising in view of the overwhelming tendency of hospitals to produce regimented patterns of care, which negates the personal needs of individual patients. Primary nursing represents the effort to reverse that trend.

It may be that the patient does not require nursing in the community. The hospital primary nurse may hand the patient over to another 'key worker', e.g. domiciliary physiotherapist or social worker, who will then take over meeting the patient's principal need. In some circumstances, where no particular help is needed at home, primary nurses in hospital might retain their contact with the patient.

Sometimes we found that patients going home were not in need of any particular help. But we made it known that we were available if advice was needed. Occasionally patients will ring up and ask to speak to their primary nurse if a problem crops up and the patient is not sure who to approach. We can either deal with it or put them in touch with the appropriate person.

Primary nurse

20.   How Do You Introduce Primary Nursing?

Planning the change has been emphasised in the earlier chapters. Having read some of the questions, the reader might well be induced to ask, 'Well, how do *I* do it?' The following is a progress report which draws together some of these strands:

How I Implemented Primary Nursing – a Ward Sister's Approach.

The Early Stages

- I developed my own knowledge and self-awareness as a ward sister and found a 'vision'. I researched everything on primary nursing and examined the beliefs and the present practice on the ward.
- I compared our philosophy and practice with that of primary nursing.
- I educated myself by reading articles given to me by other colleagues and visited other staff who were already implementing primary nursing.
- Articles about the topic were gathered from nursing journals, books, etc.
- We talked with colleagues in other wards and in other hospitals to gain as much information as possible.
- I reviewed our understanding of the philosophy of primary nursing to make sure that I had a clear picture of what my goals were (i.e. by exchanging views with more senior and experienced colleagues, teachers, etc.).
- Primary nursing conferences and study days were attended.
- I sought advice and guidance from other nurses, especially from those who had already implemented primary nursing and who had more information and experience.

continued next page

continued

- The pitfalls, disadvantages and obstacles I was likely to encounter were identified and taken into consideration in the clinical area of a busy acute medical ward.

The Vision

- Once I felt confident and secure, and had a strong, clear picture of my goal, I felt that I had to communicate this to the rest of my ward staff. They too had to share the same vision and philosophy and strong motivation with regard to primary nursing for it to be successfully implemented on the ward. Everyone from nursing auxiliary to staff nurse had to think and progress in the same direction.

  In order to increase the staff's motivation, eagerness and willingness, and to develop and share the same beliefs, I spent time on the following aspects:

  (i)   The simplicity of primary nursing philosophy was discussed, i.e. the roles of a primary nurse, associate nurse and care assistant were defined. We planned ways that these roles could be co-ordinated together in a team to promote individualised nursing care.

  (ii)   Time was taken at every opportunity to chat to staff at breaks, while making beds and during simple nursing procedures, stressing the ways in which the new philosophy (primary nursing) could be applied practically.

  (iii)   Slowly, once the term 'primary nursing' was familiar on the ward to day and night staff and to doctors, etc., we had formal talks on the ward. Staff from other primary nursing wards were invited to come and talk to us about 'how they did it'. Each nurse on the ward participated in discussion and questioning.

  (iv)   We established regular ward meetings after 8.30 p.m. in order that night staff could be present.

  (v)   Regular meetings were held with trained nurses to explore the importance of the accountability and responsibility of primary nurses and associate nurses.

  (vi)   Enrolled nurses were given the choice of being primary nurses after all the responsibilities involved were explained. They all declined and were quite happy to become associate nurses.

  (vii)   The tutorial staff and others sought to explain to staff the importance of accountability and responsibility and the type of vocabulary and documentation to which we would have to adapt when keeping care plans at the patient's bedside. The importance of confidentiality was discussed.

continued next page

continued

(viii) The nursing officer was involved in our plans to implement primary nursing as we needed the support and understanding of management. Close liaison with the nursing officer, in terms of the problems encountered, e.g. the off-duty rota, lack of trained staff, etc., was vital.

(ix) In order to stimulate staff, study days were arranged at other hospitals for members of staff to attend in order to bring back fresh ideas and information. It was important to keep them interested and involved in preparation.

(x) I sought to maintain communication with all members of staff, especially night staff.

Separate meetings were held with nursing auxiliaries, enrolled nurses and staff nurses together to gain their ideas and views and to listen to their anxieties.

(xi) Each member of staff was interviewed and asked personally if he or she felt happy about working on a ward practising primary nursing. Advantages were highlighted in order to be positive and encouraging. Particular attention was paid to those who were unsure, not interested or lacking in knowledge.

(xii) The importance of all grades of staff was reinforced, and the significant roles of associate nurse, care assistant and primary nurse were clearly defined.

Creating a Primary Nursing Climate

Once I felt that the staff had a thorough understanding and positive view of primary nursing, we began to choose teams:

24	4 RGNs	4 ENs	4 NAs

= 6 patients each (on average)

- Originally, groups were organised by the ward staff, but as the skill mix is extremely important, some teams were changed to prevent personality clashes or conflicts, to avoid other management problems and to balance expertise.

- The off-duty rota was done by me at first in order to make sure that there was always a primary nurse working opposite to an associate nurse, and that care was being maintained by the same team.

- The staff had to be involved in the off-duty planning with the rule that each was 'covered' by the other. Requests had to be kept to a minimum as the priority was to ensure that each group of patients always had their primary or associate nurse on duty.

- Marker boards were placed on the ward, where, weekly, each trained

continued next page

continued

nurse was responsible for writing about an aspect of primary nursing. The comment was left on the ward for another week in order that everyone could read it. The response was very good as each member was actively involved, and they enjoyed the frequent turnover of fresh information.

- Visitors were encouraged to come to the ward and exchange ideas with staff.
- Books and leaflets were available for everyone to read.

The Final Preparation

- Doctors were involved at the regular ward sessions. Each primary nurse became responsible for the ward round of her own group of patients (four bays of six) and for their admission and discharge programme. There was a deliberate ploy to avoid sisters doing a full ward round and to encourage them to refer to the appropriate primary nurses. Other staff, such as the ward clerk, also had to be made aware that a telephone call, visitor or any other patient problem should be referred to the appropriate primary or associate nurse. Referring everything through the ward sister (the usual way of doing things) is incompatible with primary nursing.
- Photographs of the nurses accompanied the nurse's name at the bedside.
- The primary nurses, associate nurses and care assistants were identified to each patient. Name badges were supplied which included the nurse's role, e.g. senior primary nurse/ward co-ordinator.

NB   It was very important for me to hand over the authority and to take a step back and allow the staff to make the final decisions. The sister role changed drastically to that of support, teaching and guidance. The staff had to understand this too. I had to create a new role. Asking the primary nurse to arrange ambulances and to work with the consultant was a conscious effort on my part, and I had to concentrate on staff development and see myself as a resource. I tried to help, advise and support every member of staff, including the night staff, who were involved in all the new activities. I had regular meetings with them.

Finally

Don't be too firm about the time schedule – take the plunge and do it!

21.   Is the Primary Nurse the Patient's Advocate?

It is part of each nurse's role to act on behalf of patients where they are unable or unwilling to do so themselves. It may mean that the nurse helps to take forward a complaint from a patient, or uses the nursing role to help others in the multidisciplinary team to reflect upon the consequences of decisions being made which affect patients, or perhaps the nurse transmits the patient's wishes to others. Such instances are examples of nurses acting as a patient's advocate.

However, it is important to remember that nurses may not be the only advocates for patients. Others in the multidisciplinary team may also see this as part of their role. Furthermore, it may be difficult in some circumstances for the nurse to act as an objective and dispassionate advocate precisely because he or she is involved with the patient as a primary or associate nurse, or is affected by restrictions of the employing organisation. As with autonomy, so also may there be limits to advocacy. In recognition of this, many settings have developed systems to ensure that patients have other advocates available to them. Organisations such as MIND and Age Concern, for example, are often involved in advocacy schemes – helping to put forward patients' views or act on their behalf. There can be advantages to patients in having other advocates such as these, because they are not directly involved in, governed or paid by, the health organisation in which patients are, to some extent, a 'captive audience'. As a 'professional friend' (Peplau, 1952) there may be many occasions when the nurse can act as the patient's advocate, and this can be a powerful force for ensuring that patients' rights and quality of care are upheld. At other times it may be more appropriate for others to take on this role. Clearly, there are advantages for patients if they can have access to a range of people able to act in their best interests.

22. Is Primary Nursing only Workable in 'Special' Units like Nursing Development Units?

As was suggested earlier, primary nursing has been introduced into all manner of settings through the country. It was certainly under way before the Nursing Development Unit (NDU) concept gained ground in the UK in the early 1980s. A full exploration of the concept of NDUs is beyond the scope of this text, and much has been written about them recently (e.g. Salvage, 1988b; Wright, 1988b, 1992; Vaughan, 1992). NDUs undertake a whole range of planned changes, of which primary nursing may be but one. There are currently about 300 NDUs in the UK; the number of settings which are primary nursing, whether in hospital, nursing home or community, is many times greater than this.

23. What about Part-time Staff and Bank Nurses?

Staff who have working patterns such as these can be fully involved in primary nursing. The hours worked and familiarity with the setting will place some limitations on the roles which can be occupied. Whether or not the part-time nurse works as a primary nurse must be determined by the same factors that affect any other nurse, namely:

- His or her willingness to do so.
- The possession of the requisite knowledge and skills.
- The opportunity to meet the principles which underpin primary nursing, i.e. the authority (built on autonomy and accountability) to assess, plan, deliver and evaluate care for a caseload of patients. This is coupled with the need to be in a position to ensure that care is *co-ordinated* with other staff, and carried through *comprehensively* by taking account of the contribution of patients, relatives and others. It is this last point that may cause some difficulty for the part-time nurse. To be effective, the primary nurse must have sufficient contact with patients to assess their needs and

administer some of the care. But to exclude somebody because they work less than, say, 32 hours a week is too crude an instrument.

A judgment has to be made on the above criteria, taking into account the length of time that patients remain in one place.

A part-time nurse could be a primary nurse for a patient who is only on a ward or unit for a few hours, for example in day case surgery. The patient's presence in the setting may be briefer than the time the nurse spends there. Similarly, where patients have longer term needs, the part-time nurse may be able to act as a primary nurse. The patient is still there each time the nurse is at work, enabling a continuous working relationship to develop. The ability to maintain continuity of care is the deciding factor.

24.   Does Primary Nursing Work only with 'Long-stay' Patients?

Although the definition of primary nursing stresses 24-hour accountability this does not mean, of course, that the patient has to have 24-hour contact with the nurse or be in need of care for 24 hours or more. In Chapter 1 and question 17 a number of references were made to work indicating that primary nursing has been implemented in every nursing speciality. The concept of the 'named nurse' standard in the Patient's Charter (DoH, 1991) reinforces the view that wherever a patient is receiving nursing care in the health system, then it must be possible to identify the nurse responsible for that care. For example, the nurse who gives a short episode of care to a patient in an accident and emergency, outpatient or theatre department may take the role of primary nurse for that episode – even though the contact time with the patient is very short.

Primary nursing seems feasible for quite short periods of care. Wicker (1990) and Yuen (1993), for example, discuss its application in operating theatres and outpatients,

Higginson (1991) in a day hospital and Davies (1993) in an accident and emergency department.

Primary nursing may seem more problematic not with the very long or short-stay patients, but with those who fall in between! Principal causes of difficulties are nurses' shift and holiday patterns. Some common anecdotes tell of patients entering and leaving hospital but never meeting their primary nurse. It may be that:

- The admitting nurse is not the primary nurse, but explains to the patient when they may expect to see him/her.
- A system of patient allocation is used for the first few shifts until it is clear how long the patient is likely to stay in one setting; e.g., in an intensive care unit, a standard defined by one group of nurses requires that a primary nurse is allocated once the patient's condition has stabilised and it becomes apparent that the patient is likely to stay longer than 24 hours.
- If a patient's care is of short duration, but overlaps two nursing shifts, one nurse may agree to act as primary nurse, delegating the remainder of care to a colleague who will ensure the patient's safe discharge or transfer. Alternatively, they may be able to work 'flexi-time' (increasingly common in some settings) to remain with the patient until care is completed. Yet again, it may be more appropriate to allocate a nurse each shift with each taking responsibility for their own period of care.

A degree of flexibility is needed to adapt primary nursing to different settings and circumstances. It is important that teams of nurses choose the best approach in the patients' interests. Clearly the development of primary nursing and the input of the primary nurse is going to vary with the opportunities for patient contact. The application and meaning of primary nursing will not be quite the same in a long-stay mental health unit as it would be in an operating theatre. The essential principles of identifying the nurse's role and accountability will remain the same – the application will vary. Variations there will be, but they will be variations on a theme.

25.   Is There a Difference Between the Primary Nurse and the 'Named Nurse'?

There are a number of organisational approaches to the named nurse principle (Wright, 1993), and primary nursing is one of these. The primary nurse who takes overall responsibility for the patient's nursing care is the named nurse. Therefore the primary nurse/named nurse roles are one and the same.

26.   In the 'Key Worker' System, Who Is the Primary Nurse?

Where patients are cared for under the 'key worker' system, the key worker is usually the one who co-ordinates the rest of the team and is the one whose role best fits the patient's clinical needs at the time. For example, if a patient is being cared for by a nurse, speech therapist, doctor, clinical psychologist and dietitian, and his or her dominant need is for clinical psychology, the clinical psychologist would probably be the key worker. The primary nurse would be the one responsible for the nursing component of the patient's overall care. However, if the patient's main needs concerned nursing care, the nurse could be both primary nurse and key worker.

27.   What Happens if the Primary Nurse Is Absent, Goes on Holiday or Is 'Off Sick'?

A number of possible options are available, and much will depend on the anticipated length of absence of the primary nurse. The most important issue is that patients, relatives and other carers are made aware of any changes, e.g.:

- An associate nurse in the team acts as primary nurse, with another primary nurse to act as supervisor and mentor. (It may also be appropriate in some circumstances as a useful developmental step for some nurses in preparing for the primary nurse role.)
- The patient is allocated to a new primary nurse, e.g. by adding to his or her existing caseload if this is possible.
- Another nurse acts as primary nurse temporarily (see question 1 in this chapter on the use of the ward sister/ charge nurse role as an example).

It is important that any changes, whether permanent or temporary, are clearly explained to all concerned. Nurses who work well as a team (essential to primary nursing) are able to manage this problem without causing confusion to the patient and affecting the continuity of patient care.

28. If Every Primary Nurse Is Looking After His or Her Own Patients, Who Co-ordinates the Whole Team?

Once again, a number of different approaches are available which will depend very much upon the nature of the team, local circumstances and resources. There is strength in the argument that where teams of nurses are working together, being able to identify one person who can co-ordinate the activity of the teams, resolve problems, etc. is helpful to not only patients and nurses, but other staff and visitors. Black (1992), for example, has identified some of the key aspects of the co-ordinator's role, including:

- Allocating nurses to patients based on the relative dependency of each caseload.
- Relaying information between nurses.
- Answering general enquiries on the telephone.
- Attending ward rounds when the primary or associate nurse cannot be present.

In some settings the ward clerk/administrative assistant roles have been developed to include these functions

(Pearson, 1988a). In others, they may be the role of unit or team leader, or ward sister/charge nurse. Sometimes the role may be shared between the team members, with one person acting as co-ordinator for each shift (see also 'off duty' in question 8).

Many questions arise over primary nursing, and hopefully, some of these will have been answered in the preceding pages. However, there is an old adage, as the Joni Mitchell quote at the beginning of this chapter suggests, that there is no education like experience. Having grasped the vision, it is up to each nurse and each team of nurses to pursue it in their own way.

CHAPTER 5

Helping it to Happen – the Roles of Manager and Educator

Prometheus, by his free will, undertook and carried out his plan, though he knew very well the consequences of his action. He had other alternatives, but he chose the nobler one and committed himself to his decision, which was to help men do better by making them masters of their minds.

Vassiliki Lanara
Heroism as a Nursing Value

In previous chapters, it has often been noted how the change to primary nursing must come from nurses themselves. However, it has also been stressed that it cannot be left to the clinical nurses alone. They too have needs, most importantly for that supportive climate that enables them to 'get on with it'. This chapter explores some of the characteristics of the support which primary nursing needs, and how the manager and educator can contribute.

THE MANAGER'S ROLE

How can the manager facilitate primary nursing? The following case study from a nurse manager illustrates many of the principal elements of the manager's role:

First and foremost, I had to avoid the feeling among the staff that I wanted to push it (primary nursing) through. Indeed I had many uncertainties myself. How much would it cost me? Would care get better? Would the staff be happier? So I needed to think through and get information on a lot of those issues myself first. I saw my role as waiting for each ward to be ready for primary nursing, then moving in with the support when they needed it.

To be brief, some of the points of my input included the following:

- Giving time for the staff to develop at their own pace.
- Helping the staff to review the skill mix so that it would be appropriate to primary nursing. For example, my unit was heavily staffed with nursing auxiliaries – almost 80%; over time as they left I replaced them with trained staff. Currently this is now 65% trained staff – quite an about-turn, and I'm aiming for 80%. Of course there are fewer people about, but the qualities and qualifications of the staff are that much greater. By and large, I found that you could replace every 10 auxiliaries who left with about 6 trained staff for about the same cost.
- Providing resources, e.g. help with redesigning stationery, photographs, notice boards, etc., and all the peripheral things that nurses seem to need as adjuncts to primary nursing.
- Keeping the staff levels as stable as possible, including night duty, and avoiding borrowing of staff unless absolutely essential.
- Keeping an 'open door' policy so that staff could see me when needed. Also, 'walking the patch'! – being seen in the clinical areas, helping when necessary, listening to staff and their problems and involving them in decisions. A non-autocratic approach is essential.
- Helping to co-ordinate meetings of the unit's staff.
- Using praise and encouragement to reinforce the staff in their efforts, making a point of complimenting people on good work and letting them know when a positive comment or report has been made.
- Enabling the staff to participate in further development courses, working with educators and facilitating 'networking'.
- Offering advice and counselling based on my experience, and acting as an outside 'problem solver' to be used by the ward staff.
- Appraising the staff and guiding their individual development and wishes.
- Monitoring sickness and absenteeism levels, and keeping an eye open for signs of stress arising.
- Monitoring the quality of care; as care was clearly improving, according to our quality assurance results, making sure the staff knew the results.

continued next page

continued

- Involving the ward sister/charge nurse in recruitment/interviewing so that nurses chosen are more likely to fit in with the team and share similar values.
- Supporting all the staff, but the sister/charge nurse in particular, for it is they who can feel most stressed as they relinquish power and delegate responsibilities.
- Relinquishing power myself! – letting the staff have more direct control over their budgets, skill mixes, off-duties, etc.
- Being a master juggler of the staffing establishment and my budget! Primary nursing had to be included amongst my overall objectives.
- Participating in 'selling' primary nursing to other managers and members of the multidisciplinary team, and at a wider level in the health authority, so that it becomes official policy.
- Accepting myself that I must adapt to a raised level of assertiveness and self-awareness among the staff.
- Being wary of giving the staff conflicting signals, i.e. it's no good telling the staff, 'OK, get on with it, be autonomous', and at the same time expecting them to obey my orders without question. To a greater or lesser degree, depending on his existing style, the manager in primary nursing has to undergo changes too. You have to be prepared to explain your actions and help the staff to understand your own role so they don't feel that you are interfering with or controlling them.
- Stepping in with support when needed, even when they have made mistakes. Be realistic about primary nursing; it won't make everything perfect overnight.

There are many ways in which the manager can support primary nurses, but the above would be my 'top twenty' to start the ball rolling, and keep it going.

Just as the ward sister or charge nurse sets the style or climate of a ward, so the nurse manager can set the climate for a whole unit. Managers, too, need to be risk-taking, creative people in order to foster such values among their staff.

Price Waterhouse (1988), Buchan and Seccombe (1991), McLure et al (1983) all indicate that the manager has a key role in promoting job satisfaction for staff. In so doing, he or she does much to resolve recruitment and retention problems. Involving the staff in decision-making, listening to the difficulties and helping to resolve problems are crucial elements in creating a satisfactory climate for the staff. At the same time, if primary nursing puts nurses in a position to nurse in the way they would like (inability to do this is a strong dissatisfaction to nurses – Price Waterhouse, 1988), another opportunity to enhance staff recruitment and retention arises.

Manthey (1990) believes that it is a principal purpose of all managers and others in leadership positions to empower their staff. 'Leaders empower staff' so that each can fulfil their potential and act with maximum freedom and autonomy within their roles. This involves, as the above case study suggests, investing in staff development and support and letting go of many of the rigid militaristic controls which some managers seek to adopt. In empowering staff, managers demonstrate their leadership skills and, in doing so, make their own jobs easier. A team of staff who are clear about their goals, their roles and responsibilities, and are supported and developed to carry them through, are much less difficult to manage than an army of people who need constant supervision and control. It is possible to be a leader in nursing without being a manager. For example, many nurses who work in consultancy or advisory capacities, or who act as executives on Trust boards, may have little managerial control over staffing and resources. However, their contribution to the total quality of care may be considerable through the leadership, inspiration and role modelling they offer to others. Their authority is sapiential – based on wisdom and expertise in their speciality. Such authority is difficult to ignore, for it can influence the whole purpose of the organisation and underpins shared governance of decisions about patient care at all levels. Thus nurses can retain significant power and influence in the health care system without necessarily having a managerial role.

Although it is possible to be a leader in nursing without being a manager, it is not possible to be an effective manager without being a leader. Those in nursing management positions need leadership skills which inspire, motivate and empower their staff. The need to develop nursing leadership has come much more to the fore recently (NHSME, 1993; Rafferty, 1991) and the number of organisations offering leadership programmes is increasing. There appears to be growing recognition that nurses at clinical level need effective clinical and professional leaders if they are to be effective in their work themselves. Leadership skills need to be actively fostered in nursing and a variety of techniques – formal development programmes, clinical supervision, partnering with good role models, and so on – can be used. The leader/manager is a potent force for nursing development.

JOB DESCRIPTIONS

These can be completely redesigned on the lines of primary nursing. Alternatively a simple modification outlining the role occupied could be added in agreement with the staff. Clinical grading is another (thorny) issue in relation to this. Depending on the specific requirements of the role, the primary nurse must be allocated at least E/F grade, while C/D would seem most appropriate to the associate nurse. The manager has to make decisions on these issues at each stage, and in particular establish the appropriate mix of skills and grades with the ward team (see Appendix).

The creation of a stable, satisfied workforce should be the key goal of any nurse manager. It is no less essential in primary nursing.

EDUCATIONAL SUPPORT

The demands made of the role of the primary nurse require a programme of continuous education. This, it might be argued, should be the case for nurses anyway. However, there are additional and immediate aspects in primary nursing. The newly qualified nurse is rarely equipped to be launched ready-made into primary nursing. Whether, in the light of Project 2000, this situation will change remains to be seen, as it will, in any case, take many years for the effects of a new preparation of nurses to work through the system.

The appropriate role for the newly qualified nurse should be that of associate nurse. In this role she can develop her skills, learning particularly from her primary nurse colleagues. On our unit we find that at least 6 months preparation is essential before the nurse is ready to take on her own permanent caseload.

Clinical nurse specialist

Of course, nurses have their own professional responsibility to keep up to date. However, it is the role of the manager in primary nursing to enable the staff to get the further development they need, and the role of the educator to provide it. Particular areas, of course, are the needs to enhance communication and problem-solving skills, as well as to deepen the understanding of the therapeutic value of nursing. Nurses also need to become aware of the consequences of greater autonomy and accountability and to explore the value system that they are using that underpins their day-to-day practice:

Because of the need to heighten awareness of primary nursing issues among the staff, we designed a 2-week course, provided on site for them, and led by the clinical specialist, covering the following main topics.

The therapeutic basis of nursing

A part-time course for registered and enrolled nurses providing information and updating on current issues in clinical nursing:

1. The value of nursing, its essence and actions in helping and healing.
   Partnership and companionship.
   Advocacy.
2. Nursing models – what they are and their importance to practice.
   Creative thinking in nursing.
3. The nursing process – putting the model into action through problem solving.

continued next page

continued

Different approaches.
Problems with care plans.
4. Primary nursing.
   Organising care to promote patient-centred practice.
   Setting up primary nursing,
5. Primary nursing II – primary nursing in practice.
6. Primary nursing III – evaluation and accountability.
7. Changing nursing – the application of change theory to nursing practice; developing the skills of being a change agent.
8. Therapeutic nursing; 'hands on' care.
   The nurse's helping role.
   Complementary therapies – their relevance to nursing.

Clinical nurse specialist

The sample course outlined above was subsequently developed and considerably expanded, and now forms the basis (Wade, 1992) of a formal postgraduate course on the subject. Many courses had to be developed to meet ENB and the UKCC Code of Professional Conduct standards. For example, a few one-hour sessions on aromatherapy and massage are inadequate to provide the knowledge and skill for safe and competent practice. Sometimes it is possible to use external courses that have been validated by local colleges, universities and other reputable professional bodies. Quilligan (1992) outlines the special preparation that is needed to develop 'partnership' skills. Smith and Atkinson (1992) describe a special training package they developed to help enrolled nurses 'who want to take on the challenge of primary nursing'. It is worth noting that much of the development of nurses in primary nursing focuses on developing their expressive skills – those related to communicating with, teaching and comforting patients. Some of the complementary therapies (e.g. reflexology, therapeutic touch, therapeutic massage and aromatherapy) have also been useful in enhancing the nurse's abilities in 'touching' patients and contributing to the overall notion of nursing as a healing or therapeutic act.

> We set up a 'complementary therapies group', invited guest speakers each
> month and learned to practise various therapies with each other. We found
> them helpful in improving our awareness, for example, of the importance of
> touch and our abilities to do it more effectively.
>
> *Senior primary nurse*

Courses and workshops, however, should not only concentrate on content, but also on method. Experiential
techniques, role play, and so on, are all essential to develop
greater awareness and assertiveness among nurses, and to
enhance their communication skills.

It is also important that those nurses developing primary
nursing have a chance to meet with others doing likewise
(i.e. 'networking'). Both managers and educators can
facilitate this at local, regional and national level.

> We organised 'primary nursing peer support group' meetings on the unit.
> These were a great source of getting together, reinforcing ideas, sharing
> problems and getting mutual support. The manager also provided funding
> so that some of us could attend the primary nursing network meetings
> organised by the King's Fund, both in London and regionally.
>
> *Primary nurse*

It is particularly important that possibilities of providing
'on-site' education are explored, so that it appears relevant
to the staff's day-to-day practice. Some of the following
points need to be considered:

- Is a support team or teacher available to work with the
  staff in the clinical setting, e.g. the nurse manager,
  clinical teacher or tutor, or clinical nurse specialist?
- Part-time as well as full-time courses need to be provided. Some staff may wish to attend in their own time;
  otherwise the manager needs to support 'time off' as far
  as possible.
- Courses and other formal development programmes are

only part of an overall education strategy. More imaginative techniques can be added, which have been receiving much more support and attention recently. These include clinical supervision and the use of reflective practice (Schön, 1987; Johns, 1990; Butterworth and Faugier, 1992; NHSME, 1993). In primary nursing it is possible to create the 'clinical laboratory' (Infante, 1985) where staff can test out new roles and new ideas in a climate that is safely managed for both themselves and their patients.

- Development should be available to all staff. This includes untrained staff as well. The role of the care assistant, for example, can be woven into courses for nursing auxiliaries. Primary nurses also need to develop skills in leadership, co-ordination and management of the team.
- Staff development opportunities also need to include aspects of nursing leadership and management. Some primary nurses need to evolve into the general managers and senior nurse managers of the future.
- Multidisciplinary workshops, etc., may also be needed to raise awareness of primary nursing among colleagues.
- Staff from the college of nursing can assist by supporting the staff in the clinical area by providing facilities in the school for nurses for workshops and seminars, and by organising speakers and workshop leaders.
- The student nurse should be prepared in advance about primary nursing, particularly in preparation for working in areas where primary nursing is practised.
- Access to literature, library resources, etc., is essential either in the school of nursing or in the clinical area, and preferably in both.
- Special arrangements for access to courses, literature, etc., should be made available for night staff and part-time staff.
- Distance learning packages can be designed for staff who may have difficulty in getting access to formal courses (especially night staff and part-time staff).
- Staff development meetings can be held to enable the

staff to identify their own learning needs. These can also emerge at regular career counselling sessions. It might be helpful if, in any primary nursing unit, at least one senior nurse, clinical specialist or consultant nurse is delegated this function.

> It wasn't just a question of gaining knowledge. We found that primary nurses also needed to become more aware of themselves, of their communication skills, and of their potential as 'change agents'. We devised an intensive 'survival skills course', covering all these kinds of topics, and made considerable use of role play, group work and experiential techniques to heighten awareness and develop skills and coping strategies.
>
> *Consultant nurse*

Whether staff development is provided on or off site will largely depend upon the resources and personnel available. Local colleges and universities can be helpful where there are limitations in the health authority. Inevitably, where funding resources are limited, some staff might have to meet costs themselves. However, in some settings, staff have been able to enhance their resources by various fund-raising techniques (Wright and Purdy, 1988).

EMPOWERMENT

Empowerment is currently a much-used word in health care. It underpins policies such as the Patient's Charter (DoH, 1991) a principal aim of which is to empower the users of the health care system to be aware of the rights and standards which are available to them. Once knowledge of the service has been acquired, the patient is better equipped to make sure that his or her needs are met. Here empowerment is based on knowledge, and nurses appear to have a crucial role in this process. Indeed the implementation of primary nursing in the UK appears to have been a force for empowerment of nurses. By challenging established ways of thinking about and organising nurses, primary nursing seems to have 'moved nursing's thinking on' (Melia, 1990) – itself part of an empowering process. Nurses, working as partners in care in the primary nursing system, can use their role to ensure that information is given and that patients are aware of the rights and standards which should be met, and what action to take when they are not.

Similarly, if leaders/managers in the system fulfil their role of empowering staff, this includes development and knowledge-giving to enable staff to function more effectively.

There are, however, a number of other implications from this empowerment process. While there appears to be general acceptance that empowerment is a 'good thing', nurses need to be wary that it does not become a trendy slogan, to which much lip service is paid but with little action in reality. Nurses themselves, for example, need empowerment if they are to fulfil their role of empowering patients. Having then empowered both the staff and the users of the service, how is this received?

Empowered patients and staff assert themselves, ask difficult questions, make demands on resources. The effect of empowering nurses does not stop at the doors of the ward or when the nurse goes home leaving a team of colleagues behind. The personal growth and awareness that comes along in the wake of empowerment may mean that nurses not only challenge the health system and colleagues who work with it, but also established relationships and ways of doing things in the wider world.

Empowerment is not just a nursing and health care issue, it is a matter with potential ramifications in all aspects of life. The education and empowerment of nurses in primary nursing is also a women's, race and equality issue. There are over 600 000 nurses in the UK, 90% of whom are women, many from black and ethnic minority backgrounds. It does not take too much effort to imagine the implications not only for nursing or health care but for society as a whole if 600 000 empowered nurses are unleashed!

Kramer (1974) has argued that the preparation of nurses

tends to produce a variety of different types of nurses, among them the 'rutters' (nurses who simply get along with their work and do not challenge the established order of nursing) and the 'bicultural troublemakers' (nurses who learn to survive within the organisation, yet become a force for change). Primary nursing, it seems, requires many more of the latter – nurses who can be creative, knowledgeable doers (Pearson and Vaughan, 1986). Producing more nurses of this calibre requires managers and educators to help them, even with the knowledge that life with more 'troublemakers' may be less smooth! It needs a shift in the service sector (to accept that it has a duty to develop its staff, when it is not already doing so). The education of nurses cannot be abrogated entirely to the college of nursing. In essence, writes Cox (1991), managers of nursing services at all levels work 'from the mindset that *effective management is growing people*, rather than controlling people'. The climate that the leader/manager creates 'allows the staff to blossom, to reach their potential and to realise their unique contributions to the team as a whole'. They 'realise the pivotal role they play in the quality of care and the development of staff, know firsthand what it means to be a leader – creating a healthy workplace'.

At the same time, the teachers of nurses themselves might have to examine their practices. There is a need to accept the challenge of change (ENB, 1987b), to become active change agents themselves. The primary nurse is in the business of changing nursing and changing people's lives on day-to-day basis. This cannot be done without the kind of management and educational support described in this chapter.

CHAPTER 6

Review and Conclusion

Make voyages! – Attempt them!
– There's nothing else

Tennessee Williams
Camino Real

So far, the authors have sought to describe what primary nursing is, and what important features underpin it. Issues related to day-to-day operation of primary nursing have been discussed to show how it might work in a variety of settings. Clearly, from the preceding chapters the authors have considerable enthusiasm for and commitment to primary nursing; the experiences of them and their patients suggest that there are many positive attributes which far outweigh any difficulties encountered.

DOES IT WORK?

Evidence for or against primary nursing is very varied. Much has been written about it, but often from an anecdotal and subjective standpoint. Research, where it has been conducted, is alleged to have many flaws. Young et al (1981) and Giovanetti (1987) have conducted extensive surveys of published research and other papers on primary nursing. More recently Black (1992), who co-ordinated the King's Fund Centre's Primary Nursing Network project, and Ersser and Tutton (1991) have collated a considerable amount of the research on primary nursing. The majority of the evidence on this basis is undoubtedly in favour of primary nursing for the following reasons:

- The patient feels more secure and satisfied as the nurse–patient relationship develops.
- The developing relationship increases job satisfaction for nurses.
- Nurses recognise that they can make judgments acceptable both to themselves and to patients.
- Nurses gain a clearer definition of their role in the multidisciplinary team.
- A sense of involvement with patient and family is gained by the nurse, with a resulting heightened sense of responsibility for care.
- Students' and trained nursing staff's sense of learning increases.
- Nurses feel more secure in their professional function.
- Continuity of care is greater; there are fewer errors and patient complaints.
- Nurses develop their skills as teachers, with both patients and colleagues.
- Patient care is more likely to be given as planned if the person planning care is also the care-giver.
- Some reports suggest that, overall, the quality of care is improved, especially in relation to attention to patients' families, patient teaching and discharge planning.
- Use of equipment and of stores and commodities is improved.
- Fewer complaints and more patient contact produces more trusting nurse–patient relationships.
- Clarification and resolution of patients' problems is made easier through more awareness of the patient's needs.
- Group cohesion among nurses improves (although some nurses have reported increased competitiveness).
- Patient care becomes easier and more efficient (although some nurses have suggested that the close

personal contact may make nursing care more strenuous and exhausting).

- Contact and understanding with medical staff increases (although some doctors dislike not having 'sister' in overall control).
- Overall costs are reduced, especially in relation to more efficient use of resources and deployment of staff.
- Methods of documenting care improve.
- Nurses are better able to identify the 'gaps' in their knowledge and skill and identify their own learning needs.

The effects on patients and relatives of the introduction of primary nursing

I recently completed a project entitled 'The Primary Nursing Approach' as part of the ENB 941 course (Care of Elderly People). To help me to summarise and evaluate the effects of the introduction of primary nursing on a rehabilitation/continuing care ward, I carried out a small-scale survey on the effects of primary nursing on 15 patients and their relatives.

I found that all patients and relatives were in favour of primary nursing. Results suggested that relatives understood the role of the primary nurse, and an overall comment was that they felt this aspect of giving care was a better way of nursing their relatives.

Comments from the patients were very rewarding, such as:

'It's like being looked after by my own family', 'I like having my nurse looking after me – I always look out for her because I know she looks after me and knows me better than anyone else'.

From the relatives' point of view the results were summarised as follows:

'Questions can be asked directly to the primary nurse who knows her patient inside out, and answers are obtained almost immediately, so fears and anxieties are allayed and confidence is assured'.

'It's advantageous to be able to speak to the same person caring for my relatives all the time – if I have a problem or am worried about something, I can talk to the primary nurse or associate nurse and problems are sorted out much more quickly'.

Individual comments from the patients including the following:

'It's nice to have the same person looking after me – getting me up in the morning and putting me to bed at night'.

'You get used to your own special nurse and she gets used to you too – she understands my problems better than anyone else.'

continued next page

continued

> 'I love my primary nurse'.
>
> Results from the relatives' questionnaire showed that they were all in favour of primary nursing and felt that their relatives received a better quality of care on the primary nursing ward when compared to the acute ward from which their relative had been transferred, which practised conventional patient allocation/team nursing.
>
> Relatives' comments including the following:
>
> > 'The patients seem to respond better towards their own special nurse – it's good to be able to discuss their care with the same people all the time – I can think of no disadvantages'.
> >
> > 'Questions can be asked and answered so much more quickly and confidence is assured at all times – there can only be advantages for this way of nursing patients'.
>
> The summary reinforced our view that primary nursing can be seen as not only more rewarding and fulfilling for the practising primary nurse giving the care required, but also as a more satisfying, therapeutic and reassuring way of receiving care from the patient's point of view.
>
> *Primary nurse*

Whether it be larger scale projects such as those of Marram (1976), Shukla (1983), Giovanetti (1987) or Black (1992), or smaller scale ones such as that cited in the case study above (Wills, 1988), there seems to be a large body of evidence expressing positive views of primary nursing. This evidence continues to accumulate, and more British research is now emerging. Much of this is challenging some assumptions about primary nursing. Lidbetter (1990) found educational benefits for students in the primary nursing system. Savage's (1992) work indicates that nurse–patient relationships were more likely to be closer in a primary nursing ward but noted how this relationship was successfully determined 'less by individual nurses and more by the resources available'. Mead (1990b) has illuminated the difficulty in teasing out the essential discriminating features between different organisational methods, such as team nursing, primary nursing and patient allocation. Malkin (1993) could find no significant difference between primary and non-primary nurses' levels of intrinsic job satisfaction or intentions to stay in nursing. Primary and non-primary nurses were found to gain job satisfaction in different areas of work. Reed's (1988) survey, on the other hand, suggested that greater job satisfaction was obtained by primary nurses. Meanwhile, the Audit Commission (1991), McMahon (1990b), Carr-Hill et al (1992), NWRHA (1992), Pearson et al (1992), Bond et al (1991) and MacGuire (1991) have all produced evidence, in varying degrees of strength, supporting the application of primary nursing, particularly in the fields of improving the quality of patient care and staff collaboration, communication and satisfaction.

With such an enormous range of alleged benefits, despite some reservations, it is little wonder that a primary nursing 'bandwagon' got under way (Wright, 1988a) in the UK. Beset by many troubles, it seems that the search by nurses to find their panacea is not a new phenomenon. Throughout nursing history, innovations have been taken up with wild enthusiasm and applied with great energy, but with little consideration for the evidence of real or imagined benefits or disadvantages. Is primary nursing falling into this trap?

Certainly, if primary nursing were to go ahead solely on the basis of incontrovertible evidence, it would never have happened at all.

Giovanetti (1987) and Black (1992), for example, cite many methodological inconsistencies in the research they surveyed: lack of definition of primary nursing, doubts about whether like is compared with like, size of samples, and so on. MacDonald (1988) notes how much of the available literature is of North American origin and thereby questions its applicability to the UK nursing culture and organisation of health care. Arguments ensue as to whether it is cheaper or more expensive to implement primary nursing. Shukla (1983) found evidence for increased staffing costs, while Binnie's (1987) work suggests these may be less. Variables, then, have to be considered, e.g. skill mix and experience of staff, and grades of pay may cloud the issue.

Giovanetti (1987) also notes how 'calling a nurse a primary nurse and assuring continuity of patient assignment, for example, did not automatically result in increased authority, responsibility and accountability'. Manthey (1980), meanwhile, argues that merely organising primary nursing is of itself no guarantee of improved quality of care, although it should put nurses in a position where they are empowered to do better: 'Many people have mistakenly equated the concept of a system of care delivery with the concept of quality of care. The quality of nursing service in primary nursing can be good or bad, comprehensive or incomplete, co-ordinated or spasmodic, individualised or standardised, creative or routine'.

Throughout this text it has been argued that it is insufficient simply to reorganise groups of nurses and their skill mix. It is necessary also to examine the *values and attitudes* that underpin their practice and the *knowledge and skill* with which they practise. These factors are as crucial to primary nursing, and as inseparable from it, as the way in which nurses are deployed.

A fundamental principle of primary nursing is that, in reorganising nurses, there is a concurrent planned approach to question, develop and, where necessary, change the whole philosophy and practice of nurses and their care. The commitment to primary nursing is nothing less than this.

Bowers (1989) succinctly summarises and posits a number of other issues in relation to primary nursing. It may merely be a symptom of the desire for more professional status by nurses and part of a long history of attempts by nurses to wean themselves away from the control of others, notably doctors and latterly general managers. He raises questions about autonomy and accountability – how can nurses exercise these when others are constantly telling them what to do? How can they be responsible for the quality of care when so much of it (e.g. the provision of resources) is dependent on others? How far does primary nursing represent a desire by managers to control costs and nurses? (Managers would find it easier to identify an individual accountable nurse.)

Meanwhile, primary nursing might put at risk the cohesiveness of the ward team or uncover 'conflicts between doctors and nurses' (Bowers, 1989).

Bowers further argues that there is a political dimension in the UK to the adoption of primary nursing:

> 'The rise of Thatcherism and the new right is having an impact on nursing in the UK. Large public bureaucracies are now believed to be inefficient. Structural changes are being made in order to make the system appear more efficient. Primary nursing fits hand in glove with these notions' (Bowers, 1989).

In the rush towards primary nursing, a bandwagon had been set in motion that tended to swamp the many doubts around it. As has been argued in earlier chapters, the traditional ward team may be less than the cohesive unit it is imagined to be, and it is the experience of all the contributors that team spirit tends to increase, not diminish, with primary nursing. Issues of accountability and autonomy have produced gross dissatisfaction with care, from both nurses and patients, in the past. Primary nursing is a manifestation of the effort to resolve these dilemmas. Meanwhile, the 'doctor–nurse game' (Stein, 1978), based on the accepted power structure between the two, leaves much to be desired.

'The doctor–nurse game' describes the relationship between doctor and nurse as an elaborately ritualised façade. In this way, nurses are able to manipulate the doctor's decision without overtly undermining his status or authority. Each partner has to be acutely sensitive to the non-verbal and cryptic cues given by the other. Each learns the game through a long process of socialisation as each gains experience in their respective fields. Stein says:

> 'The nurse is to be bold, have initiative and be responsible for making significant recommendations, while at the same time she must appear passive. This must be done in such a manner as to make her recommendations appear to be initiated by the physician'.

Thus, open disagreement between doctor and nurse is to be avoided at all costs and the nurse can communicate recommendations without appearing to make a recommendation statement.

This strategy appears to help both doctor and nurse defuse what could otherwise be a very conflict-ridden area of their work. However, this restricts an honest dialogue and may stifle initiative. Nursing knowledge and skill is cloaked, and appreciation of its true value may be lost. It is not clear how the end product of this social 'pas-de-deux' between doctor and nurse benefits the patient. If primary nursing upsets the status quo between doctors, nurses and other disciplines, perhaps this is long overdue. Where a truly collegial relationship already exists, primary nursing will probably enhance, not diminish, relationships, for it will reinforce, not detract from, the clarity of the role of each discipline. Stein has recently revisited his earlier work and finds many changes. Nurses appear to have been forging new roles, asserting themselves and clarifying their identities and contribution to health care. As a result, the old doctor–nurse game is becoming increasingly less relevant. Some doctors have responded positively to the revised collegial relationship with nurses, others have reacted with hostility and confusion (see Chapter 4, question 15). Stein et al (1990) note: 'Although some physicians long wistfully for the return of the hierarchical doctor–nurse relationship and resist the changes that are occurring, the forces of change are inexorable and universal'.

If reorganising nursing care falls into the trap set by politicians and managers, there must indeed be caution in developing primary nursing. However, as has been suggested throughout this text, primary nursing is more than a mere restructuring of the hierarchy or a redeployment of actions and responsibilities. It is a whole new way of thinking about and carrying out nursing. To see it merely as reorganisation is to underestimate and misunderstand it.

To attempt to interpret and evaluate it in strict scientific terms also has its limitations. Professional judgment can be dismissed as subjective and therefore invalid. The living, qualitative relationship that can exist between nurse and patient can be dismissed as mere emotion, untranslatable into cost-effective terms. If primary nursing is in part a philosophy of care:

> 'then we must proceed with philosophic inquiry into the nature of primary nursing. In the absence of this inquiry, attempts at measuring the effects of primary nursing using scientific means are premature, for they will be as ineffective in the future as they have been in the past. Philosophic questions are not answerable through the scientific method. Whatever the source is of these problems, they must be addressed. To ignore them is to assume that research in nursing will not provide a sound basis for making decisions about ways and means of improving nursing care' (Giovanetti, 1987).

POWER AND PROFESSIONALISM IN PRIMARY NURSING

Many writers, such as Bowers (1989), seem to suggest that primary nursing is a symptom of professionalisation in nursing. It is a sign of the desire to become more powerful by being a profession. On this issue it is right to be cautious. If primary nursing encourages development of an élitist power group of nursing, all that will have happened is for power over patients to be transferred from one power group to another. Will nursing then fall into this traditional mould of professionalism, or is there an alternative for a nursing profession based on different values – the values inherent in primary nursing?

The difference here is a fundamentally important one, and it is an issue to which nurses in practice must address themselves in the onward rush to professional status. Should nursing be a profession? Nursing exists to serve the health needs of clients and patients. How can it organise itself so that the service position to the consumer is ensured, so that high standards of practice are maintained and developed? How can the construction of a monstrous professional megalith be avoided, which may in the end expend more energy in preserving its own integrity and value than in acting as the guardian of and supplicant to the patient's rights?

The interests of nurses and the interests of patients are often one and the same, and both should be allies in the fight to resist the interests of the powerful few, especially in a time of increasingly élitist medicine and shrinking resources. Often dazzled by the white heat of the advance of medical technology and the power and prestige of medicine, the consumers' opportunities to exercise power and control over their own health needs are minimised. Nurses are befuddled by confused gender hierarchies (male/doctor dominance, female/nurse subservience) and trapped by the altruism of their calling. If only Florence Nightingale had trained her nurses in assertiveness instead of military obedience to dogma and authority! Miller (1979) argues that altruism has created a paradox for nursing. It may serve society but it does little to help the nurse. In addition, the nurses' subservient role hinders them in their fight as an advocate of the patients' rights, when the patients themselves may not have the power to fight for themselves. Oakley (1984) notes that people who belong to subordinate groups such as nurses and women 'tend to be socialised into a psychological pattern which emphasises dependency, passivity, subservience, and thinking about other people's welfare'. The socially dominant groups, e.g. men or doctors, learn qualities of independence, initiative, control, domination and putting their own welfare and development ahead of other people. The issues involved are highly complex, and this book has already begun to address itself to some of them in examining the way in which nurses organise themselves, their role in the process of change and their relationships with other health workers.

Nurses in the practice of primary nursing must be in the vanguard of questioning the application of professionalism to nursing. A powerful élite commanding high status and salary would have to be smaller than at present; significant rises in pay could not be given to what is currently a massive, homogeneous group. Would this mean an even smaller body of trained nurses governing the activities of the untrained? Or might a system develop where the label 'professional' is only applied to relatively few nurses who have spent a longer period in vocational training (as doctors do)? Contrast this with the current system, which trains a nurse for 3 years, then considers him or her capable of full nursing responsibilities.

An awareness is developing among nurses of the value of nursing and of advancing their practice, not merely as a reflection of the narcissistic mirror that medicine offers, but in the mirror offered by the patient based on the level of satisfaction. The advanced 'professional nurse' is both teacher and healer, enhancing skills and knowledge, but in so doing offering these to patients so that they are in control of their own health and not subject to a market dominance or monopoly by nurses.

It is a source of regular debate at conferences and in the nursing press as to whether or not nursing is a profession. Perhaps this debate is a reflection of an inherent insecurity in nurses as a result of their oppressed status. As Greer (1991) points out, 'As long as they like themselves, they will not be an oppressed minority. In order to like themselves they must reject trivialisation by others of who and what they are'. One of the threads running through primary nursing is the assertion of the value of nursing.

The purpose of primary nursing is to provide the medium through which nurses can attain the highest quality of patient care. Can nurses do this without falling into the traditional professional mould? Perhaps nurses need not look to established definitions of a profession, but re-cast it in their own image. Professions are often described as élite groups with a clearly identifiable body of knowledge which they exclusively control and which they sell, at a price, to clients. Nursing could hardly be judged as a profession on these criteria.

Perhaps the issue is, should nurses judge themselves in this way? Do nurses wish to have power [which as Hugman (1991) argues is what professionalism is all about] over others, however benignly it is used?

There is nothing wrong with nurses associating themselves with certain aspects and behaving 'professionally', for example, using expertise for the service of others. Indeed, in the public domain, the word professional is very loosely used – referring most commonly to people who show skill, knowledge and dedication in what they do. Perhaps nurses should judge themselves a little less by how others define a profession.

Such judgments may reflect a lack of self-confidence. In addition, George Bernard Shaw's assertion that professions are 'conspiracies against the laity' reminds us that the behaviour of such groups is not always in the wider public interest. Perhaps nurses can redraw the boundaries of professionalism for themselves. Nurses can determine their own path and reject the models set by others. The foundations are already there – we speak of working as partners in care, of sharing and caring, and of being a public service.

Indeed, nursing is the only discipline which makes the theme of 'caring' the prime directive of its existence. Other groups suggest they 'care', but only nursing sets this at the head of its occupational goals and raison d'être.

Professions often espouse the concept of service to others but in reality the client is at the mercy of their expertise – the roles are reversed. It is the client who is powerless, who is the servant. If Patients' Charters and nursing principles are to have any value, they must be about the professions giving their power to empower the patient. Nurses are ideally placed to take on this role and thus redefine the nature of professionalism in an image jointly determined by themselves and those who have need of them.

In acquiring knowledge and skill, they have a greater goal than professional aggrandisement. It is to share this knowledge and skill with those who have need of it, to be a force for empowerment of others and not over others. Thus, by working in a way which 'turns the servant into the master through the use of expertise' (Wilkes, 1981), nurses can bring a new meaning to the concept of professionalism. In so doing nurses can reject the definitions set by others, which serve only to trivialise them and their work. Instead, nurses can have the confidence to be different, and to be of real and lasting value to the community.

A fundamental philosophical shift of emphasis is required, which must be largely the task of nurses in practice. 'Power' to many nurses is almost a dirty word, but they must take it to act both on a political and personal level to serve their clients. Nursing must be a new kind of powerful profession, sharing, not hiding, knowledge and skill – open and working with clients as partners, not closed and controlling or dominating them. Having grasped power, nurses must then pass it right into the hands of patients, by working with them as partners or companions. Nurses would thus give a new character to the behaviour of a profession. Whatever form the changing face of nursing takes, however far it becomes 'professional', nurses in practice and those who support them must build the safeguards that ensure that nursing is the instrument of the patient, not the patient the instrument of nursing. This is one of the fundamental challenges of primary nursing.

CONCLUSION

There are many ways forward in nursing, and primary nursing is but one of them. It is a method of organising care based on certain essential philosophical assumptions about nursing. It is not just a means of redeploying the nursing team, but a whole way of thinking about nursing, which identifies it as valuable, creative, skilful and therapeutic in its own right. Primary nursing puts the trained nurse in a position to be accountable for, and autonomous in, giving the total nursing care of a patient or group of patients. The care is co-ordinated by that nurse, who may be assisted by others acting as his or her associate, in a comprehensive pattern throughout the patient's stay in his or her setting, and fully involves the patient, the family and other carers and members of the multidisciplinary team in the nursing of the patient. The essence of primary nursing lies in the nurse–patient relationship, and elements (autonomy, accountability and so on) which nurses incorporate into their roles. Many of the aspects discussed in this book help primary nursing to be implemented – going out of uniform, patient access to nursing notes, the use of personal cards, introducing complementary therapies – but they are trappings tagged on to the essence. It is interesting to note that where nurses have implemented primary nursing, they have also tended to venture into other areas of change. Whether primary nursing stimulates more changes or is a product of them is debatable. Certainly, it seems to be a common phenomenon that where primary nursing is happening, then a number of other elements tend to be tagged on as part of a general review of care and attempts to make it more personal. In that sense primary nursing may not just be a product of Pandora's box, something that nurses do once they have been liberated in other ways. It may be a Pandora's box itself, letting loose a wide range of innovations once primary nursing itself is under way.

To develop nursing in such a way may seem hopelessly unrealistic to many nurses. Beset by problems of resources and reorganisation, it is little wonder that primary nursing may be little more than a vision to many – a utopian dream that would be so nice, it's true – if only we had the staff, or supportive managers, or decent facilities!

Indeed, there are challenges facing nursing now – the increased pressure to 'ration' health care (Bowling, 1992), the increased emphasis on care in the community, the rise of the 'patient focused hospital' with its 'multi-skilled' workers (RCN, 1992), the continued restructuring of the health service with even greater pressure for 'cost-effectiveness', and questioning the role and value of qualified nurses. Factors such as these make it essential, more than ever before, that nurses are very clear about their roles and why nursing is valuable. Nurses will be called upon more and more to meet these challenges: they may either adapt and turn them to their advantage, try to resist them, or be swept aside as irrelevant to the new health agenda.

Primary nursing has the potential to help nurses clarify their roles and be very certain about the value of nursing practice – especially in a health care system which increasingly demands the ability to convince others, the purchasers, that nursing is worth buying. Primary nursing can help to empower nurses so that they can expand their role, whether it be in mastery of the 'patient-focused' initiative or developing nurse practitioner roles or nurse-managed beds. As with all changes, there are many threats but also many opportunities.

The journey on the road towards primary nursing is fraught with difficulties. It needs complex and long-term plans to overcome them. Should we wait for research before we proceed? After all, primary nursing is not *proven* to be effective, and wouldn't it be safer just to stay as we are? Primary nurses and those who support them must be voyagers, for they venture out, often into uncharted territory it is true. If we always waited for evidence, for research, for clear maps to guide the way, we would never go anywhere. We would be afraid to turn the next corner for fear of the uncertainty that lies beyond it. This book has been an attempt to chart the territory of primary nursing a little more clearly.

The hopes in primary nursing may be branded as unrealistic. Those who promote it may be accused of not living in the 'real world'. Where primary nursing has succeeded, it has often been against considerable odds. Those nurses have not lived in an unreal world; they have simply set about creating a new reality for themselves, however long – sometimes years – it has taken.

The status quo does not seem to be an option. The Health Service, for example, has endorsed primary nursing as a way forward (DoH, 1989; NHSME, 1993), recognising that there remain in nursing many dark corners of inadequate care (Martin, 1984; Health Service Ombudsman, 1986–1993). New initiatives are needed to improve standards of care. Encouragement from these and other quarters (or from managers who might see it as a means to greater control in cost-cutting) needs to be treated with caution. Otherwise there is a risk that this support transforms into a rod with which to beat the clinical nurses (you *must* do primary nursing because the Department says so!!). Primary nursing needs extensive preparation, continued support and time, perhaps many years, to grow.

All nursing before primary nursing was not bad, and all that follows it will not inevitably be good. Primary nursing is not a panacea. It will not cure nursing's ills overnight. It will not suddenly produce patients who are loving and co-operative, it will not instantly remove interdisciplinary conflicts and it will not make nurses immediately kind to one another. All nurses will not suddenly become expert communicators, night staff will not quickly lose their sense of isolation and nurses will not cease to go 'off sick'. What primary nursing will do is enable nurses to confront these and many more issues of conflict in nursing and, more importantly, empower them to do something about them. Primary nursing may produce conflicts, but many of them are problems we have long covered up. Tackling them is long overdue.

Primary nursing will only work where nurses are ready and willing to take on board their accountability and autonomy, to work with colleagues in a relationship of equals, and to share care with patients and other carers as partners and companions. It will only work when managers and educators take on their rightful role as supporters of clinical nursing, not just its controllers. The more you control, the less you create.

If success does not come as fast as we would wish, it is right to remember that it is not all our fault! If you are not instantly achieving in primary nursing, it may not be your problem, so do not feel guilty. Nurses often take the guilt of their failings onto their own shoulders. It should be remembered that others play a part too – those who are unhelpful or obstructive. In this case, when guilty feelings arrive, perhaps it is worthwhile off-loading them to the real source of the problem.

Meanwhile, value and cherish what you do that makes care personal. There is much that can be done to make life better for patients that does not depend on primary nursing.

Primary nursing is part of a long process of change in nursing, in which nursing and its inherent values are reawakened and its territory rediscovered and redefined, part of a movement of renewal in nursing which Salvage

(1990) has defined as 'new nursing'. If nurses do not do this, others will – and not necessarily to the benefit of patients. Primary nursing is a way of thinking and working with patients that challenges established practices and undermines outmoded customs. Nurses in primary nursing are the termites of the nursing establishment. However, all this must be for the practical benefit of patients, otherwise it is mere intellectual tennis. It is the challenge to nursing to work with patients as people, test out our values and redefine our practice.

It is the call for the nurse to work with 'my patients', to provide the humane personal help and healing, which the patients want from 'my nurse'. Pursue your vision!

Sample Job Descriptions for Primary Nursing

Please note that these are examples of job descriptions only. Modifications will need to be made for permanent night duty staff, where the night nurse is likely to be an associate nurse yet carry additional supervisory, clinical and managerial responsibilities [e.g. night nurses (associate) are graded on scales from D through F to reflect these factors].

JOB DESCRIPTION 1

Role: Care assistant

Grade: A

Responsibility to: Deputy UGM/head of nursing services (Unit I) through the senior nurse manager (Care of the Elderly and Nursing Development Unit)

Accountable to: Senior primary nurse/primary nurse

Job summary:
The principal aim of the care assistant's role is to support the primary nurse/associate nurse in the delivery of nursing care. This may be by directly assisting the nurse with his/her caseload of patients or by helping with general ward organisation.
The post-holder will:

- Assist the primary/associate nurse as required in the giving of care, within the unit's agreed guidelines for the activities of the care assistant.
- Assist with general orderliness of the ward.

- Carry out delegated non-nursing activities to assist the primary nurse/associate nurse.
- Assist with appropriate aspects of nursing care under supervision.
- Contribute to maintaining the ward's agreed philosophy, aims and objectives.
- Keep the primary/associate nurse informed of observations relating to patient care.
- Work with colleagues to help co-ordinate nursing and other activities on the ward.
- Follow agreed unit and health authority policies in relation to personal and patient safety.
- Keep up to date by attending to personal development, attending appropriate lectures, etc.
- Maintain the confidentiality of the patients and their care.
- Work as part of the team to promote a climate on the ward conducive to learning and high standards of patient care.

This job description is intended to give a broad outline to the function and responsibilities of the care assistant and may be updated at regular intervals.

A job description is not a rigid or inflexible document but acts to provide guidelines to the duties expected while in post.

This job description will be reviewed and amended in the light of changing professional demands.

JOB DESCRIPTION 2

Role: Associate nurse

Grade: C

Responsibility to: Deputy UGM/head of nursing services (Unit I) through the senior nurse manager (Care of the Elderly and Nursing Development Unit)

Accountable to: Senior primary nurse/primary nurse

Minimum qualifications: State enrolled nurse

Job profile:
The associate nurse works under the direction of the primary nurse to assess, plan, implement and evaluate the nursing care of a given caseload of patients.
The post-holder will:

Clinical

- Give care to patients under the direction of the primary nurse.
- Assist with assessing, planning, implementing and evaluating care.
- Liaise with the primary nurse to co-ordinate the overall plan of care.
- Accurately document nursing care.
- Work according to the ward's agreed philosophy, nursing model and objectives.
- Work with the primary nurse to produce a therapeutic ward environment for patient care.

Educational

- Keep up to date with current nursing practice.
- Accept responsibility for maintaining professional development and identify own learning needs.
- Help colleagues by passing on expertise to others and participate in the overall plans of the wards to promote learning.

Management

- Assist in the supervision of care assistants.
- Co-ordinate his or her own activities with the rest of the ward to ensure achievement of the ward's objectives.
- Work according to unit and health authority policies and the UKCC Code of Conduct.
- Promote the safety of self, colleagues and patients at all times, in relation to equipment, the ward environment, etc.
- Take part in other duties as agreed within the unit's policies.

Research

- Make use of appropriate research findings in nursing practice.
- Co-operate with colleagues with research projects and the evaluation of care.

A job description is not a rigid or inflexible document but acts to provide guidelines to the duties expected while in post.

This job description will be reviewed and amended in the light of changing professional demands.

JOB DESCRIPTION 3

Role: Associate nurse

Scale: D

Responsibility to: Deputy UGM/head of nursing services (Unit I) through the senior nurse manager (Care of the Elderly and Nursing Development Unit)

Accountable to: Primary nurse/senior primary nurse

Minimum qualifications: RGN/SEN with relevant post-qualification experience

Job profile:
1. The post-holder is responsible for assisting with the assessment of care needs, and the development of programmes of care, and/or implementation and evaluation of these programmes.
2. The post-holder is expected to carry out all relevant forms of care without direct supervision and may be required to demonstrate procedures to, and supervise, qualified and/or unqualified staff.

The post-holder will:

Clinical

- Be a safe practitioner.
- Liaise with and provide relevant information to other members of the multiprofessional team.
- Assist in the facilitating of a therapeutic environment that meets the needs of the patients.
- Take responsibility for a caseload of patients in the absence of the primary nurse.
- Co-ordinate the patient's care with the primary nurse.
- Assess, plan, implement, evaluate and document care in association with the primary nurse.
- Work with colleagues to promote the development of the ward's philosophy, nursing model and agreed clinical objectives.
- Work with colleagues to develop clinical expertise and high standards of nursing practice.

Research

- Demonstrate a commitment to developing his or her own research skills.

- Be receptive and supportive towards the research plans of others.
- Contribute to the application and evaluation of current research findings.

Management

- Occasionally take responsibility for the management of the ward and patient care in the absence of a more senior nurse.
- In the absence of a more senior nurse, be responsible for the co-ordination of all activities within the ward.
- Help to maintain positive working relationships with the multidisciplinary team.
- Ensure the promotion of safety, well-being and interests of patients, staff and all visitors to the clinical area.
- Be aware of the district health authority policies and procedures and carry these out in the clinical area.
- At all times follow the Code of Professional Conduct as laid down by the UKCC.

Educational

- Under the guidance of senior sister/charge nurse (scale G), identify own learning needs.
- Assist in the facilitating of a learning environment conducive to the acquisition of further knowledge and skills.
- Contribute, where appropriate, to the development of teaching strategies, taking into account the needs of staff and patients.
- Liaise with colleagues to co-ordinate the approach to the development of staff in the ward.

A job description is not a rigid or inflexible document but acts to provide guidelines to the duties expected while in post.

This job description will be reviewed and amended in the light of changing professional demands.

JOB DESCRIPTION 4

Role: Primary nurse

Scale: E

Responsibility to: Deputy UGM/head of nursing services

(Unit I) through the senior nurse manager (Care of the Elderly and Nursing Development Unit)

Accountable to: Senior primary nurse/senior sister/charge nurse (scale G)

Minimum qualifications: RGN plus at least 6 months post-registration experience and evidence of further development in the speciality with particular reference to preparation for primary nursing.

Job profile:
1. The post-holder is responsible for the assessment of care needs and the development, implementation and evaluation of programmes of care.
2. The post-holder is expected to carry out all relevant forms of care and may regularly take charge of a ward or equivalent sphere of nursing in the absence of the person who has continuing responsibility. The post-holder is expected to supervise junior staff and will be expected to teach qualified and unqualified staff, including basic and/or post-basic students, where applicable.
3. The post-holder is required to take responsibility as the primary nurse for a defined group of patients and may act as an associate nurse in the absence of a colleague. He/she works with minimal supervision in the assessment of all relevant care needs and in the development, implementation and evaluation of programmes of care.
4. The post-holder is expected to participate fully in quality assurance initiatives, with particular emphasis on a 'customer first' approach.

The post-holder will:

Management

- Take responsibility for the management of the ward and patient care in the absence of a more senior nurse, with the aim of setting the highest possible standards.
- In the absence of a more senior nurse, be responsible for the co-ordination of all activities within the ward or equivalent sphere.
- Help to create and maintain positive working relationships within the multidisciplinary team.
- Ensure the promotion of safety, well-being and interests of the patients, staff and all visitors to the clinical area.

- Be aware of the district health authority policies and procedures and carry these out in the clinical areas, and ensure that all junior staff follow these policies and procedures.
- At all times follow the Code of Professional Conduct as laid down by the UKCC and ensure that all staff within this sphere of responsibility also follow the code as laid down.
- Contribute to monitoring the performance of staff within the sphere of responsibility and report to the senior sister/charge nurse (scale G).

Clinical

- Demonstrate clinical excellence.
- Liaise with, and provide relevant information to, other members of the multiprofessional team.
- Assist in the supervision and monitoring of nursing practice under the guidance of the senior sister/charge nurse (scale G).
- Assist in the facilitating of a therapeutic environment that meets the needs of the patients.
- Carry a clinical caseload as a primary nurse, and act as an associate nurse for colleagues where appropriate.
- Contribute to the development of the ward's philosophy and nursing model.
- Contribute to meeting the agreed clinical objectives for the ward.
- Work with senior colleagues to develop further clinical expertise and develop soundly based nursing practice.

Research

- Demonstrate commitment to developing their own research skills.
- Be receptive and supportive towards research plans of others.
- Contribute to the application and evaluation of current research into care.
- Participate in appropriate research/evaluation studies on the ward.
- Contribute to the documentation of the activities of the ward.

Educational

- Contribute as a counsellor and adviser to the learners and other ward staff on matters related to care of the elderly, in the absence of a more senior nurse.
- Accept personal responsibility for identifying his or her own learning needs and professional development.
- Assist in the facilitating of a learning environment conducive to the acquisition of further knowledge and skills.
- Contribute to the development of teaching strategies appropriate to the needs of staff and patients.
- Be prepared to accept the role of a preceptor/mentor.
- Liaise with all colleagues in a teaching capacity to ensure an overall co-ordinated approach to staff development.

A job description is not a rigid or inflexible document but acts to provide guidelines to the duties expected while in post.

This job description will be reviewed and amended in the light of changing professional demands.

JOB DESCRIPTION 5

Role: Primary nurse/sister/charge nurse

Scale: F

Responsibility to: Deputy UGM/head of nursing services (Unit I) through the senior nurse manager (Care of the Elderly and Nursing Development Unit)

Accountable to: Senior primary nurse/sister/charge nurse (continuing responsibility – scale G)

Minimum qualifications: RGN plus at least 2 years appropriate post-registration experience including evidence of further development in the speciality.

Job profile:
1. The post-holder is designated regularly to take charge of a clinical area of nursing in the absence of the person who has continuing responsibility.
2. The post-holder is responsible for the assessment of care needs and the development, implementation and evaluation of programmes of care, without supervision, and may be required to teach other nursing and non-nursing staff.

3. The post-holder will be a primary nurse who may also act as an associate nurse for colleagues.
4. The post-holder will be required to act up for the G grade.
5. The post-holder is expected to participate fully in quality assurance initiatives with particular emphasis on a 'customer first' approach.

The post-holder will:

Managerial

- Take responsibility for the management of the clinical area in the absence of the sister/charge nurse (scale G), with the aim of setting the highest possible standards, following the agreed guidelines laid down in the ward's philosophy of care/ aims and objectives.
- Help to create and maintain positive relationships between all groups involved in the welfare of the patient.
- Be responsible for the co-ordination of all activities in the absence of the sister/charge nurse (scale G).
- Ensure the promotion of safety, well-being and interests of the patients, staff and visitors to the clinical area.
- Communicate as necessary to all staff the district health authority policies and procedures and carry these out in the clinical areas, and inform all junior staff of any changes to them so that they follow these policies and procedures.
- At all times follow the Code of Professional Conduct as laid down by the UKCC and ensure that all staff within their sphere of responsibility also follow the code as laid down.
- Assist and support the sister/charge nurse (scale G) in planning staff duty rotas to meet the requirements of the unit and clinical areas.
- Monitor the performance of staff within their sphere of responsibility and report to the sister/charge nurse (scale G).

Clinical

- Demonstrate clinical expertise and act as a positive role model.
- Act as a clinical adviser to the multiprofessional team.
- Be responsible for supervising and monitoring nursing practice under the guidance of the sister/charge nurse (scale G).
- Facilitate a therapeutic environment that meets the needs of the patients.

- Contribute to the development of the ward's philosophy and nursing model to promote the aims of personal nursing care.
- Act as a primary nurse and co-ordinate the care of a given caseload of patients from admission through to discharge.
- Participate in pursuing the agreed ward objectives in the promotion of high standards of care.
- Strive to ensure that all nursing practice is based on sound rationale.
- Accurately pursue and document the assessment, planning, implementation and evaluation of nursing care.

Research

- Demonstrate a commitment to developing research skills in themselves and junior staff.
- Be receptive to the research plans of others and encourage full co-operation with all the staff.
- Assist in the application and evaluation of current research findings.
- Participate in appropriate research/evaluation studies on the ward.
- Contribute to the documentation of activities/evaluation of care on the ward.

Educational

- Participate in the teaching and development of all grades of staff on the ward.
- Act as mentor/preceptor where appropriate.
- Identify own learning/development needs and take steps to pursue objectives.
- Liaise with the senior primary nurse/ward sister/charge nurse to co-ordinate teaching/learning activities on the ward.
- Contribute as a counsellor and adviser to the learners and other staff on matters related to the care of the elderly.
- Facilitate a learning environment conducive to the acquisition of further knowledge and skills.

   This job description is not a rigid or inflexible document but acts to provide guidelines to the duties expected while in post.
   This job description will be reviewed and amended in the light of changing professional demands.

Management

- Be responsible for the continuous management of the clinical area of nursing over 24 hours, with the aim of setting the highest possible standards, following the agreed unit philosophy.
- Be responsible for budgetary control for their clinical area of nursing.
- Be responsible for the creation and maintenance of positive working relationships within the multidisciplinary team.
- Be responsible for the co-ordination of all activities within the clinical area of nursing.
- −Ensure the promotion of safety, well-being and interests of patients, staff and all visitors to the clinical area.
  −Pay particular regard to the district health authority's fire procedures.
- Act as change agent to promote innovation and high standards of practice.
- Communicate to all staff the district's policies and procedures, inform all staff of any changes to them and ensure that staff follow these policies and procedures.
- Inform the representatives of each committee, should procedures or policies require updating.
- At all times follow the Code of Professional Conduct as laid down by the UKCC and ensure that all staff within their sphere of responsibility also follow the code as laid down.
- Plan the staff duty rotas to meet the requirements of the unit, ward and patients' needs and to facilitate primary nursing.
- Monitor and appraise the performance of staff within their sphere of responsibility.
- Monitor nurse−patient dependency levels.
- Monitor staff sickness and absence and take appropriate managerial action.
- Work on day and night duty shifts as appropriate to meet the needs of 24-hour responsibility for the ward.

Clinical

- Demonstrate clinical excellence and high standards of nursing practice to other staff.
- Be responsible for supervising and monitoring nursing practice and be accountable for the same.

- Develop a therapeutic environment that meets the needs of the patients.
- Work with colleagues to set standards of clinical nursing and organise care to achieve these.
- Retain a clinical input by acting as a primary or associate nurse.
- Promote clinical activities that give appropriate participation to patients, relatives and other carers in the process of care.
- Meet clinical objectives as agreed separately with the senior nurse manager and consultant nurse.
- Identify and develop a model of nursing practice to promote the goals of personal nursing care.
- Ensure that the care of all patients is assessed, planned, implemented, evaluated and appropriately documented.

Research

- Demonstrate a commitment to developing research skills in themselves and other staff.
- Be receptive to the research plans of others and encourage full co-operation from all staff.
- Apply, where appropriate, and evaluate findings of current research into patient care.
- Carry out studies and research projects appropriate to the field of expertise.
- Identify areas of study/research on the ward, document these activities and review with the consultant nurse for wider dissemination of findings/activities.
- Develop methods at ward level to monitor standards of care in liaison with the clinical nurse specialist (quality assurance/research).

Educational

- Act as a counsellor and adviser to students and other ward staff related to care of the elderly.
- Accept personal responsibility for identifying own learning needs and professional development.
- Develop a learning environment conducive to the acquisition of further knowledge for all staff.
- Identify the training needs of all staff within their sphere of responsibility and develop teaching strategies appropriate to the needs of staff and patients.

- Be an ENB assessor.
- Accept the role of preceptor where applicable.
- Act as a role model and mentor to colleagues in the demonstration of high standards of practice.
- Liaise with other staff involved in education in the unit to provide a cohesive approach to the development of students and staff.
- Act as a clinical adviser to the multiprofessional team.

A job description is not a rigid or inflexible document but acts to provide guidelines to the duties expected while in post.

This job description will be reviewed and amended in the light of changing professional demands

References

Argyle M. (1978) *The Psychology of Interpersonal Behaviour*. Harmondsworth: Penguin.

Aschjem O., Carlsen L.B. and Markussen A.B. (1979) Primaersykepleie lever i norge, og har det ganske bra! *Sykepleien*, 66(17): 6–11, 13.

Audit Commission (1991) *The Virtue of Patients*. London: HMSO.

Audit Commission (1992) *Making Time for Patients – A Handbook for Ward Sisters and their Managers*. London: HMSO.

Benner P. (1984) *From Novice to Expert*. London: Addison Wesley.

Benner P. and Wrubel J. (1989) *The Primacy of Caring: Stress and Coping with Death and Illness*. Menlo Park: Addison Wesley.

Bergman R. (1981) Accountability – definition and dimensions. *International Nursing Review*, 28(2): 53–59.

Beyers M. and Phillips C. (1971) *Nursing Management for Patient Care*. Boston: Little, Brown.

Biley F. (1989) Treatment and care: patient participation in decision-making. *Senior Nurse*, 9(10): 23–24.

Biley F. (1991) Patient involvement in nursing decisions. *Nursing Times*, 87(36): 54–55.

Binnie A. (1987) Primary nursing: structural changes. *Nursing Times*, 83(39): 36–37.

Black F. (ed.) (1992) *Primary Nursing – An Introductory Guide*. London: King's Fund.

Blanpain J.E. (1976) Systems analysis of the nursing unit: primary nursing, a holistic approach to the delivery of nursing care. Unpublished document cited in *The Change to Primary Nursing* (1982) Hegyvary S.T. London: C.V. Mosby.

Bond S., Bond J., Fowler P. and Fall M. (1991) Evaluating primary nursing. Series of 3 papers published in *Nursing Standard*, 5(36): 35–39; 5(37): 37–39; 5(38): 36–39.

Bowers L. (1989) The significance of primary nursing. *Journal of Advanced Nursing*, 14: 13–19.

154   *My Patient – My Nurse*

Bowling A. (1992) Setting priorities in health: the Oregon experiment. *Nursing Standard*, **6**(37): 27–30; **6**(38): 28–30.

Buchan J. and Ball J. (1991) *Caring Costs – Nursing Costs and Benefits*. University of Sussex, Brighton: Institute of Manpower Studies. Report No. 208.

Buchan J. and Seccombe I. (1991) *Valuing Nurses: Pay, Careers and Working Patterns of Qualified Nurses*. University of Sussex, Brighton: Institute of Manpower Studies.

Butterworth A. and Faugier J. (1992) *Clinical Supervision and Mentorship in Nursing*. London: Chapman and Hall.

Caines E. (1990) In: Vision or nightmare? Naish J. *Nursing Standard*, **5**(12): 18–20.

Caines E. (1993) In a report. *The Guardian*, 15.5.1993, p.20.

Campbell A.V. (1984) *Moderated Love*. London: SPCK.

Carr-Hill R., Dixon P., Gibbs I., Griffiths M., Higgins M., McCaughan D. and Wright K. (1992) *Skill Mix and the Effectiveness of Nursing Care*. University of York: Centre for Health Economics.

Cassée J. (1975) *Therapeutic Behaviour, Hospital Culture and Communication*. In: *A Sociology of Medical Practice*, eds. Cox C. and Mead A. London: Collier-MacMillan.

Chilton S. (1991) A change in the right direction. *Nursing Times*, **87**(25): 44–46.

Chopra D. (1989) *Quantum Healing*. London: Bantam.

Cox S. (1991) A healthy workplace – the manager's role. *Primary Nursing*, **10**(2): 3.

Davies J. (1993) Applying the named nurse concept in an accident and emergency unit. In: *The Named Nurse, Midwife and Health Visitor*, ed. Wright S.G. (1993). Leeds: NHSME.

Dean D. (1988) *Manpower Solutions*. London: RCN.

Department of Health (1989) *A Strategy for Nursing*. London: DoH.

Department of Health (1991) *The Patient's Charter*. London: HMSO.

Dimond B. (1988) *The Law and the Nurse*. Unpublished paper, Nursing Times Primary Nursing Conference, Manchester.

Dyson R. (1991) *Changing Labour Utilisation in NHS Trusts*. Keele: University of Keele.

Dyson R. (1993) In: 'Under Fire', Friend B. *Nursing Times*, **89**(18): 19.

English National Board for Nursing, Midwifery and Health Visiting (1987a) *Circular No. MAT/28*. London: ENB.

English National Board for Nursing, Midwifery and Health

Visiting (1987b) *Managing Change in Nursing Education.* London: ENB.

Ersser S. and Tutton E. (1991) *Primary Nursing in Perspective.* Harrow: Scutari.

Finch M. (1991) The steady advance of a revolution. *Nursing Times*, **87**(17): 67–68.

Georgiades N.J. and Phillimore L. (1975) The myth of the hero-innovator. In: *Behaviour Modification with the Severely Retarded*, eds. Kiernan C.C. and Woodford F.P. London: ASP.

Giovanetti P. (1987) Evaluation of primary nursing. *Annual Review of Nursing Research*, **1**(4): 127–151.

Gooch S. (1992) Patients cannot choose prejudice. *Nursing Standard*, **6**(34): 41.

Greer G. (1991) *The Change.* London: Hamish Hamilton.

Hall L.E. (1969) The Loeb Centre for Nursing and Rehabilitation. *International Journal of Nursing Studies*, **6**: 82–83.

Hancock C. (1991a) Name that nurse! *Times Health Supplement*, **8**(11): 10.

Hancock C. (1991b) Blowing the trumpet. *Nursing Times*, **87**(34): 26–27.

Health Service Ombudsman (1986–1993) *Reports of the Health Service Parliamentary Liaison Officer (Ombudsman).* London: DHSS.

Hegyvary S.T. (1982) *The Change to Primary Nursing.* London: C.V. Mosby.

Henderson V. (1980) Preserving the essence of nursing in a technological age. *Journal of Advanced Nursing*, **5**: 245–260.

Higginson I. (1991) Applying primary nursing in the day hospital setting. *Primary Nursing News*, **2**(4): 4.

Hiscox H. (1990) Primary nursing in an ENT ward. *Primary Nursing News*, **1**(8): 3.

Hugman R. (1991) *Power in Caring Professions.* London: MacMillan.

Infante M.S. (1985) *The Clinical Laboratory in Nursing Education.* Chichester: Wiley.

Institute of Manpower Studies (1992) *Motivation, Morale and Mobility: A Profile of Qualified Nurses in the 1990s.* Brighton: IMS.

Johns C. (1990) Autonomy of primary nurses: the need to both facilitate and limit autonomy in practice. *Journal of Advanced Nursing*, **15**: 886–894.

Kafka F. (1916) *Metamorphosis* (reprinted 1974). Harmondsworth: Penguin.

156 *My Patient – My Nurse*

Karpov I. (1991) Primary nursing in Finland. *Nursing Times*, 87(17): 69–70.
Kemp J. (1992) Night-time associates. *Nursing Times*, 87(4): 63–65.
Kitson A. (1988) On the concept of nursing care. In: *Ethical Issues in Caring*, eds. Fairbairn G. and Fairbairn S. Aldershot: Avebury Press.
Kramer M. (1974) *Reality Shock*. St Louis: C.V. Mosby.
Ku Y.C. (1993) Promoting the system of 'My Patient – My Nurse'. Madrid: International Council of Nurses.
Lanara V. (1981) *Heroism as a Nursing Value*. Athens: Sisterhood Evniki.
Lathlean J. (1988) Viable reality a pipe dream? *Nursing Times*, 84(49): 39–40.
Lawler J. (1991) *Behind the Screens*. Edinburgh: Churchill Livingstone.
Lee M.E. (1979) Towards better care: primary nursing. *Nursing Times* occasional paper, 75(33): 133–135.
Lidbetter J. (1990) A better way to learn? *Nursing Times*, 86(29): 61–63.
McDermott B. (1992) Primary school. *Nursing Standard*, 24(6): 56.
MacDonald M. (1988) Primary nursing: is it worth it? *Journal of Advanced Nursing*, 13: 797–806.
McFarlane J. and Castledine G. (1982) *A Guide to the Practice of Nursing Using the Nursing Process*. London: C.V. Mosby.
MacGuire J. (1988) Does mix matter? In: *Options and Opportunities*, DHSS. London: DHSS.
MacGuire J. (1991) Quality of care assessed: using the Senior Monitor Index in three wards for the elderly before and after a change to primary nursing. *Journal of Advanced Nursing*, 16(5): 511–520.
McLure M.L., Poulin M.A., Sovie M.D. and Wandelt M.A. (1983) *Magnet Hospitals – Attraction and Retention of Professional Nurses*. Kansas City: American Academy of Nursing.
McMahon R. (1990a) Power and collegial relations among nurses on wards adopting primary nursing and hierarchical ward management structures. *Journal of Advanced Nursing*, 15(2): 232–239.
McMahon R. (1990b) Collegiality is the key. *Nursing Times*, 86(42): 66–67.
McMahon R. and Pearson A. (1992) *Nursing as Therapy*. London: Chapman and Hall.
Machiavelli N. (1514) *The Prince* (translation by G. Bull, reprinted 1986). Harmondsworth: Penguin.

Malkin K.F. (1993) Primary nursing: job satisfaction and staff retention. *Journal of Nursing Management*, 1: 119–124.
Manthey M. (1970) Primary nursing. *Nursing Forum*, **IX**(1): 65–83.
Manthey M. (1973) Primary nursing is alive and well in the hospital. *American Journal of Nursing*, **73**: 83–87.
Manthey M. (1980) *The Practice of Primary Nursing*. London: Blackwell.
Manthey M. (1988a) Can primary nursing survive? *American Journal of Nursing*, **88**: 644–647.
Manthey M. (1988b) *A Commitment to Each Other*. Minneapolis: Creative Nursing Management.
Manthey M. (1990) The nurse manager as leader. *Nursing Management*, **21**(6): 18–19.
Marks-Maran D. (1978) Patient allocation v task allocation in relation to the nursing process. *Nursing Times*, **74**(10): 413–416.
Marlow S. (1991) The right attitude. *Nursing Times*, **87**(11): 42–44.
Marram G.D. (1976) The comparative costs of operating team or primary nursing. *Journal of Nursing Administration*, **6**(4): 21–24.
Martin J.P. (1984) *Hospitals in Trouble*. London: Blackwell.
Mead D.M. (1990a) Research report: collegial relationships among primary and associate nurses. *Nursing Times*, **86**(42): 68.
Mead D.M. (1990b) *Innovations in Nursing Care: The Development of Primary Nursing in Wales*. Cardiff: Unpublished report to the Welsh Office.
Medaglia M. (1978) A coronary care unit implements primary nursing. *Canadian Nurse*, **74**(5): 32–34.
Melia K. (1990) A decade of change. *Nursing Times*, **86**(26): 33–34.
Menzies I. (1961) The functioning of social systems as a defence against anxiety (reprinted 1988). In: *Containing Anxiety in Institutions*, Menzies-Lyth I. (1988). London: Free Associate Books.
Miller J.B. (1979) *Towards a new Psychology of Women*. Boston: Beacon Press.
National Health Service Management Executive (1992) *The Patient's Charter – Guidance for Implementation*. Leeds: NHSME.
National Health Service Management Executive (1993) *A Vision for the Future*. Leeds: NHSME.

Nightingale F. (1869) *Notes on Nursing, What It Is and What It Is Not* (republished 1980). Edinburgh: Churchill Livingstone.

North Western Regional Health Authority (1992) *Ward Nursing Quality and Grade Mix*. Manchester: NWRHA.

Oakley A. (1984) The importance of being a nurse. *Nursing Times*, **80**(50): 24–27.

Otoya T. (1979) Advantages and disadvantages of team nursing: a trial at primary nursing. *Kangogaku Zasshi*, **43**: 163–169.

Ottoway R.N. (1976) A change strategy to implement new norms, new styles and new environment in the work organisation. *Personnel Review*, **5**(1): 13–18.

Ottoway R.N. (1980) *Defining the Change Agent*. Unpublished Research Paper. Department of Management Sciences, University of Manchester Institute of Technology.

Payne C. (1991) *Management Issues in Primary Nursing*. Unpublished paper. Presented to the Primary Nursing Conference: Huddersfield, June 1991.

Pearson A. (ed.) (1988a) *Primary Nursing*. London: Croom Helm.

Pearson A. (1988b) Trends in clinical nursing. In: *Primary Nursing*, ed. Pearson A. London: Croom Helm.

Pearson A. (1992) *Nursing at Burford: A Story of Change*. Harrow: Scutari.

Pearson A. and Vaughan B. (1986) *Nursing Models for Practice*. London: Heinemann.

Pearson A., Punton S. and Durand I. (1992) *Nursing Beds – An Evaluation of the Effects of Therapeutic Nursing*. London: Scutari.

Pembrey S. (1980) *The Ward Sister – Key to Nursing*. London: RCN.

Peplau H. (1952) *Interpersonal Relations in Nursing*. New York: Putnam.

Perera R. and Miller F. (1993) *Primary Nursing Teaching Package*. London: St Thomas' Hospital.

Price Waterhouse (1988) *Nurse Retention and Recruitment*. London: Price Waterhouse.

Purdy E., Wright S.G. and Johnson M.L. (1988) Change for the better. *Nursing Times*, **84**(38): 34–36.

Quilligan S. (1992) Educational preparation and support for nurse–patient partnership. *Nursing Times*, **88**(16): 78.

Rafferty A.M. (1991) *Leading Questions*. London: King's Fund Centre.

Rankin-Box D. (1993) Innovation in nursing practice: complementary therapies in nursing. *Complementary Therapies in Medicine*, 1(1): 30–34.

Reed J. (1988) A comparison of nurse-related behaviour, philosophy of care and job satisfaction in team and primary nursing. *Journal of Advanced Nursing*, 13(3): 383–395.

Reilly D. (1975) Why a conceptual framework? *Nursing Outlook*, 23(9): 12–20.

Remington I. (1989) Night rites. *Nursing Times*, 85(1): 30–31.

Roth H. (1993) Primary nursing in progress. Madrid: International Council of Nurses.

Rotkontch R. (1979) Personal communication. Cited in *The Change to Primary Nursing* (1982), Hegyvary S.T. London: C.V. Mosby.

Royal College of Nursing (1986) *The Education of Nurses: A New Dispensation*. London: RCN.

Royal College of Nursing (1992) *Task Focussed Hospitals or Patient Focussed Care?* London: RCN.

Royal College of Nursing (1993a) *Staff Side Evidence to the Pay Review Body*. London: RCN.

Royal College of Nursing (1993b) *Refusal to Care*. (Issues in Nursing and Health Series No. 18). London: RCN.

Salvage J. (1985) *The Politics of Nursing*. London: Heinemann.

Salvage J. (1988a) *Facilitating Model Based Nursing*. Unpublished paper. Nursing Models Conference, Gateshead.

Salvage J. (1988b) Nursing Developments. *Nursing Standard*, 3(22): 25–28.

Salvage J. (1990) The theory and practice of the 'new nursing'. *Nursing Times*, 86(4): 42–45.

Savage J. (1992) Keeping in touch, *Nursing Times*, 88(49): 30–32.

Sayre-Adams J. (1993) Therapeutic touch – principles and practice. *Complementary Therapies in Medicine*, 1(3): 96–99.

Schön D. (1987) *Educating the Reflective Practitioner*. San Francisco: Jossey-Bass.

Shukla R.K. (1983) An all RN model of nursing care delivery: a cost benefit evaluation. *Inquiry*, 20: 173–184.

Smith H. and Atkinson M. (1992) Enrolling for the future. *Nursing Times*, 88(16): 73–75.

Sparrow S. (1986) Primary nursing. *Nursing Practice*, 1(3): 142–147.

Stein L. (1978) The doctor–nurse game. In: *Readings in the Sociology of Nursing*, ed. Dingwall R. and MacIntosh J. Edinburgh: Churchill Livingstone.

Stein L., Watts D. and Howell T. (1990) The doctor–nurse game revisited. *New England Journal of Medicine*, **322**(8): 546–549.

Stockwell F. (1972) *The Unpopular Patient*. London: RCN.

Strong P. and Robinson J. (1988) *New Model Management: Griffiths and the NHS*. Warwick: Nursing Policy Studies Centre, University of Warwick.

Toffler A. (1973) *Future Shock*. London: Arrow.

Toshiko T. (1993) The difference of patients' satisfaction between primary nursing and team nursing. Madrid: International Council of Nurses.

Turnock C. (1990) Preparing for primary nursing. *Nursing Standard*, **5**(12): 34–36.

Turrill T. (1985) *Change and Innovation: A Challenge for the NHS*, Management Series 10. London: Institution of Health Service Management.

Tutton L. (1986) What is primary nursing? *Professional Nurse*, **2**(2): 39–40.

United Kingdom Central Council for Nursing, Midwifery and Health Visiting (1983) *Code of Professional Conduct for the Nurse, Midwife and Health Visitor*. London: UKCC.

United Kingdom Central Council for Nursing, Midwifery and Health Visiting (1986) *Project 2000*. London: UKCC.

United Kingdom Central Council for Nursing, Midwifery and Health Visiting (1992a) *The Code of Professional Conduct*. London: UKCC.

United Kingdom Central Council for Nursing, Midwifery and Health Visiting (1992b) *The Scope of Professional Practice*. London: UKCC.

Van Eindhoven J.M.B. (1979) Patient-orientated ward organisation. *International Nursing Review*, **26**: 3.

Vaughan B. (1992) Nursing Development Units – the pursuit of excellence. *Nursing Times*, **88**(31): 26–28.

Wade L. (1992) A diploma in primary nursing. *Primary Nursing News*, **3**(3): 2.

Waterman S. and Luker K. (1990) Reluctant collaborators: do patients want to be involved in decisions concerning care? *Journal of Advanced Nursing*, **15**: 971–976.

Waters K. (1985) Team nursing. *Nursing Practice*, **1**(1): 7–15.

Watson J. (1978) Patient evolution of primary nursing project. *Australian Nurses Journal*, **8**(5): 30–33.

Wicker C.P. (1990) A reassuring presence. *Nursing Times*, **86**(29): 59–61.

Wilkes R. (1981) *Social Work with Undervalued Groups*. London: Tavistock.

Wills G. (1988) An evaluation of primary nursing in a continuing care/rehabilitation ward. Unpublished survey, Nursing Development Unit, Tameside General Hospital.

Wills G. and Wright S.G. (1988) Getting to know you. *Nursing Standard*, 3(9): 32.

Wilson-Barnett J. and Carrigy A. (1978) Factors affecting patients' responses to hospitalisation. *Journal of Advanced Nursing*, 3: 221–228.

Wong J. (1979) An exploration of a patient-centred nursing approach in the admission of selected surgical patients: a replicated study. *Journal of Advanced Nursing*, 4(6): 611–619.

Woods D. (1987) *Biko*. Harmondsworth: Penguin.

Wright S.G. (1986) *Building and Using a Model of Nursing*. London: Arnold.

Wright S.G. (1987a) Consuming interests. *Senior Nurse*, 62: 24–26.

Wright S.G. (1987b) Patient centred practice. *Nursing Times*, 83(38): 24–29.

Wright S.G. (1988a) The bandwagon effect. *Nursing Standard*, 3(5): 42.

Wright S.G. (1988b) Defining the Nursing Development Unit. *Nursing Standard*, 4(8): 29–31.

Wright S.G. (1989) *Changing Nursing Practice*. London: Edward Arnold.

Wright S.G. (1992) Exporting excellence. *Nursing Times*, 88(39): 40–42.

Wright S.G. (ed.) (1993) *The Named Nurse, Midwife and Health Visitor*. Leeds: NHSME.

Wright S.G. and Purdy E. (1988) If I were a rich man. *Nursing Times*, 84(41): 36–37.

Young J.P., Giovanetti P., Lewison D. and Thomas M.L. (1981) *Factors Affecting Nurse Staffing in Acute Care Hospitals: A Review and Critique of the Literature*. (DHEW Publication No. HRP050180C). Hyattsville, USA: Department of Health Education and Welfare.

Yuen P. (1993) The named nurse in an outpatient department and operating theatre. In: *The Named Nurse, Midwife and Health Visitor*, NHSME (1993). Leeds: NHSME.

Index